Skinny Genes

Weight Gain Explained & the CURE

By Dr Phil Harley

Published by BrainSolutions
2016

Dr Phil Harley
BrainSolutions.co.uk

ISBN-13: 978-1517452582
ISBN-10: 1517452589

"The best time to plant a tree was 20 years ago. The second best time is now."

Chinese Proverb

CHAPTER ONE

Welcome section

Introduction

This is Skinny Genes. It is a book about why our genes make us fat. It is about the science behind it. All explained in an easy-to-get-your-head-around-it way. Many of us feel our waistlines are a little out of control. It is a bit of a mystery why it keeps expanding. Many of us don't understand why we think and do the things we do. It seems mysterious how waistline control is so difficult to achieve.

But it makes sense. Really it does. I will explain how and why. When you understand more, you can make better choices. These will lead to way better results. Consistently. No more yo-yo dieting. I will show you a straightforward system that you can use for the rest of your life. We will explore why your body and brain work the way they do. The way they interact to produce weight loss and weight gain. We will find out the best ways to lose weight and stay in control.

Putting on weight is not your fault. It is human nature. It is in our genes.

Putting on weight is a fault of both our biology and the world we live in today. Using this knowledge we will see how to beat the system and to regain control of your waist. You will discover how to control your body, its urges, signals and drives, rather than having them control you. No one likes to feel out of control.

Feel free to cut to the tips & nudges section. Use its action lists to get started. But do come on back, because understanding how it all fits together will help even more. After learning in the main section what makes us think, behave and act the way we do around food, the rest of it will seem easier. It begins to fall into place and all starts to make sense.

Managing your waist is about using and responding to your body intelligently.

Fuel your body well and it will look after you for many long years to come.

There are no hard and fast rules here. You are a complex biological organism made up of thousands of complex interacting systems. The interplay of these systems follows predictable patterns. These patterns will emerge throughout this book. Understanding how the body, mind and spirit work together will help you to make better choices. These better choices will help move you each and every day towards your goals.

* * *

We are all unique even though we are complex biological systems that function identically. We have our own personalities and operate slightly differently to everyone else on the planet. Although we sometimes seem to behave quite differently there are patterns which can help all of us.

Happily we are all descended from the same ancestors. Our bodies and minds have evolved over many thousands of years, shaped by the same environmental conditions. These selection pressures in survival situations are shared in our DNA. You and I share 99.9% of our genetic blueprint.

Because we are so similar, medical science can show us how we are the way we are. Science shows us how we think, behave and do the things we do. The secrets of our body, mind and spirit are no longer a mystery.

Skinny Genes is all about practical steps to manage your waist. This is very manageable. I will show you how.

If you become lost while reading this, do not panic. You don't have to understand everything in this book. It makes more sense the second time around. It's even ok if you don't find the detail interesting. Feel free to just use the checklists or even simply follow the diary. These will simply work just by following them. I've put all the rest of it in to help you to apply the best techniques that modern medicine and modern psychology have to offer. I find the details and the reasons behind what makes us tick absolutely fascinating. I hope you will too.

Survival and replication

You are a survival machine. The DNA in your cells has survived for millions of years. It has been copied billions of times. Your ancestors all survived long enough to have offspring. These offspring then survived to grow up and repeat the process. You are the latest in a long line of successful survivors who had children. **Who also survived successfully**.

You are designed to survive. You are designed to replicate. By this I mean your body and everything in it is designed to fulfil these functions. Every thought you have and every biological urge you feel are designed to drive you towards putting yourself in optimal situations for reproducing and then the survival of your genes.

If your ancestors weren't as good at surviving as their neighbours they would have been the more likely to die out. If they weren't as good at mating and having offspring as their neighbours they would have been less likely to pass on their genes and nature would unapologetically have **weeded them out.**

We are all here because our distant relatives were fantastic at surviving infancy, childhood, adolescence, seeking out a mate, having sex and then ensuring the baby went on to survive infancy, childhood and so on. That's it. There are no other traits which will do better in the world we all came from. There are no features of your body which don't serve a function towards surviving and passing on your genes. **It is not enough to simply replicate.** Your offspring need to survive to become fertile and produce successful offspring of their own.

The genes we carry in each of our cells are virtually the same as when we lived on the African plains. We are identical in our bodies and minds to nomadic tribes. It is only forty thousand years ago since we were like this. This is a blink of an eye in evolutionary terms. Only a few hundred generations separate us. Which means our genes have not had enough time to change in the last forty thousand years.

We are not adjusted for twenty-first century life.

Your genes come from a time when we lived in very hot conditions with limited food and water. We mainly gathered our food. Nuts, berries, fruit and roots. We occasionally killed large prey like antelopes, but small birds and rodents would have been more common fare. In the last forty thousand years we have domesticated animals and learned farming. We no longer rely on our small group to survive and we have food in abundance. We now cook our food so twelve hours a day doesn't need to be spent chewing, just to get enough nutrients to survive. This has freed up a lot of time. Machines have made a lot of other things easier too. We each live today in greater luxury than Kings and Queens of only a few hundred years ago.

But, we are still ruled by the same emotions and desires that powered us for life on the African plains. We eat whenever we can and our bodies rapidly lay down any excess in fat stores because the next meal might be days or even weeks away. We are driven to fit in with the group for its survival benefits. We strive to gain social status where we can and to seek out and try to mate the best possible partners to pass on our genes. This is what makes us tick.

Understanding this can help us regain control of our waists.

Making better choices

Good waist management is all about making better choices. Better choices each and every day. These choices shape our future. They shape who we are. Who do you want to be? What shape would you like to be? What choices can you make right now, today and for the rest of the day which will support you on this journey?

Making better choices about what you put in the top end will affect what your body does. You wouldn't expect a Formula One car to run very well on low grade fuel. A jet aircraft needs aviation fuel otherwise it will not fly. Your body is pretty incredible in how well it can do, even when we put rubbish in. Just imagine how much better it would be if we always put high quality nutritious food in. Imagine if we always put in just the right quantity to match the needs of our body.

This book is about showing you how to make better choices,

what those better choices are and how to stick with them once you've got the hang of it.

I hate dieting too

I hate dieting too. Diets are rubbish.

Diets are all about being deprived. We manage to lose a little weight. We feel miserable on them and end up putting it all back on again after.

Dieting doesn't work very well. You may have noticed. Lots of people succeed in the short term. But then we gain weight when the diet stops and the efforts slide. This is heartbreaking. All your jolly hard efforts gone to waist. It's all rather inconvenient that the rewards don't last. If it all goes wrong when we stop, how do we carry on? How do we stay on track and motivated? Good question. The answer is **motivation**. This need to be compelling.

You need a goal. One which motivates you and then a plan.

* * *

I don't know what will motivate you. Maybe you don't either? Knowing why you want to control your waist is key. Having your goal in mind will help you to break it down into smaller manageable steps. The technical phrase is 'chunking down'. This means making it easier to get your head around and thus more achievable in the **real** world. This will keep you focussed and moving forwards.

If there is nothing that drives you, nothing you *really* want, you are not likely to succeed. Don't waste any more of the limited number of valuable seconds we are alive on this planet reading another page. Go away.

Come back when you are ready with something that you want to achieve. Some people want to be a size fourteen. Some people want to see their kids graduate from high school. Some people want to feel good about themselves when they see themselves in family photographs. Some people want to turn heads next summer when they wear their bright red thong bikini (or mankini) by the pool on holiday (in a good way). It doesn't matter too much what your specific motivation is. It only matters that it matters to you.

Motivation can be about improving your health. It could be living longer. It could be about wanting better sex. I really don't mind what you choose but it's got to be what **you** want. Write it down. Right now. Write now. What three things do you want to be a whole load better in a year? How about five years? How about ten, twenty? Do you still want to be alive and kicking?

There is a story about motivation I like;

A man sits in the psychiatrist's chair toying with a cigarette. He says to his therapist;

"I really struggle with giving up, I mean I get the health benefits and the cost and all that, I just find that I like the smoking more, I enjoy it…"

The therapist leaps up, reaches behind him pulling a pistol from his waistband. He holds it to the man's head and screams;

"PUT THAT CIGARETTE DOWN!"

This is affectionately known as Smith & Wesson therapy. I imagine it can be rather effective.

When the motivation is big enough we can achieve nearly anything. The trick is in finding stuff that matters enough to you to want to change. Then making better choices seems a whole lot easier.

CHAPTER TWO

Is this book for me?

Who this is for

This book is for everyone. I mean everyone. We are all the same. We have been engineered to perfection over millions of years of evolution. We are amazing biological machines. Our minds are the most complex and the most advanced that we know of in the entire universe.

As a race we all share the same wiring, the same physical systems, the same genetic code and the same chemical processes at the level of individual cells. I've spent many years reading, learning and understanding all of this to put into daily practical use as a doctor. We are pretty amazing creatures.

The really great thing is that all of these systems, cells and processes have been shaped by the same environmental pressures and biological needs. This means that body and mind make sense. Human thoughts and behaviours can seem mystifying at first, but when you peer a little closer; what we think, do and even say makes a whole lot of sense.

This is extremely helpful because in Skinny Genes I will show you practical ways to manage your waist the way that you want. Today, tomorrow and lifelong.

Who this is not for

*This book **not** for anyone who doesn't want more from their life.*

*This book is **not** for those who aren't interested in how to do things better.*

*This book is **not** for anyone who is not wanting a bit of a change.*

This book is all about change. It is about how to get more from life. This book is all about making better food choices and better day-to-day decisions.

Making better choices and making better decisions will transform your life.

Managing your waist is a challenge. It is not always easy and that's ok. There are plenty of things in life that aren't easy but are well worth achieving. When you achieve something that is difficult you gain an enormous sense of well being.

Controlling your waist isn't complex but fitting it into your life can seem that way at first. If it didn't require any thought, everyone would manage it. You may have noticed that this doesn't really happen. You may also have noticed that year on year our nation is expanding. This expansion isn't showing any sign of slowing down.

In the Middle Ages they thought that you consisted of body, mind and spirit. These artificial, ancient and archaic divides resonate even today.

The body needs fuel. The mind needs to be in control. The spirit needs a sense of purpose and life direction.

We can help our **body** by fuelling it well, moving it better and using its urges, desires and feelings to provide valuable feedback on how we are doing.

We can help our **mind** by letting it understand what the body is doing. We can give the mind some sense of control over what is happening and use it to help make us feel good.

We can nurture our **spirit** by having clear goals and concentrating on the stuff that motivates us.

Connecting the body mind and spirit together helps all three parts work better, producing a synergistic sense of wellbeing.

Dr Phil Harley

How to use the book

The book has an opening section (which you could skip), followed by lots of detail about the way we are wired and why getting a grasp on this is helpful for you. It explains why dieting isn't very successful as a strategy - despite us spending millions of dollars, pounds, euros and yen each and every year on it (you may have noticed people getting rich out of this and you aren't one of them).

The book then has a section of tips and gems that other people have found really helpful and asked me to include.

To finish, we have the workbook, the diary (don't skip this - it's the best bit. If've you've got the Kindle version, really consider buying the paper diary. Using it makes a huge difference).

How does it all work? - read the information, understand how it all works (or doesn't), make more informed choices and use the workbook. Make better choices lifelong. Do it from a place of better knowledge and understanding. This is written to give you the very latest in modern medical knowledge. It uses cutting edge psychology and the best that today's scientific research has for you.

Rubbish in, rubbish out

The human body is an amazing thing which can cope with a spectacularly wide array of foods. It specialises at extracting the required parts of nutrition and excreting the rest.

You have biological priorities for every calorie you eat. You cannot change these. Fuel the brain, then survive. Have sex, look after the kids. Then lay down fat. In that order. Every time.

Our bodies need enough calories to keep our brains and vital organs functioning. We also need to move well enough to survive and reproduce. Any excess energy is laid down efficiently into our fat layers as a store for leaner times.

This amazingly efficient biological organism works for and against us. It works for us so we can put any old rubbish in and will reliably extract the protein, vitamins, minerals, vital fats and essential amino acids needed to function perfectly. It works against us only when we have an excess of energy. And most of us do. On most days.

Eat less, move more and everything will improve.

We are perfectly evolved to thrive in an environment where food is scarce and are not designed to cope with the excess of food most of us eat today. This works against us because we are so efficient at laying down fat. We lay down the cuddle around our middle to keep us alive in the food scarcity of winter. We prepare too well, this fat layer shoving us towards an early grave. Our curvy middles lead to joint destruction, make us unhappy and to add insult to injury, we don't look nearly as sexy as we used to when examining ourselves in front of a mirror. The naked truth.

Being too heavy affects the blood vessels. Hardening of the arteries contributes to high blood pressure and in turn early death and disability from heart attacks and strokes. Weight related diabetes worsens those along with giving erectile dysfunction, loss of sensation in hands and feet, amputations, blindness and chronic severe nerve pains. Weight related arthritis causes long term pain and disability, sometimes requiring joint replacement surgery. Some people can't even walk.

We are not designed well to cope with an excess of fat. Our moods suffer, we become depressed, we slow down. We tend to enjoy life less and our sex lives suffer.

More than one third of the women in the USA and the UK are

currently overweight or obese. They are much less likely to conceive and much more likely to have a miscarriage if they do. They are also at increased risk of heavy unpredictable periods. Being overweight increases the risk of nearly every cancer, including breast and womb cancer. Being overweight increases the risk of severe chest infections and increases the risk of clots in the veins in the leg (deep vein thrombosis - DVT), which can spread to the lungs (pulmonary embolus - PE) and kill you.

Currently a quarter of children in the USA and UK at the age of eleven are overweight or obese. This is a big problem, getting bigger every year. Being overweight now kills more people and causes more disability than smoking.

Being in control

We all like to feel in control. When we feel out of control we feel distressed. This is one of the definitions of stress.

If we feel out of control with what our body is doing, we don't feel good. When life gives us too many challenges and not enough resources to manage them, we feel stressed. When we have too many things to do and not enough time to do them, or they are beyond our capabilities, we don't cope very well. Not having enough money for all the things we need to spend it on is also stressful.

Many of my patients feel like this. Many feel that they can't control their waistlines and because this makes them feel bad, they comfort eat. This too makes them feel bad and they then can't cope with the other stuff that life throws at them each and every day. They aren't very happy and don't really know how to start turning it around.

This book will show you how regain control over the waistline. I will show you a plan to follow if you would like. If you stick at this and complete the diary at the end, you will regain control. If you have the e-book version, be sure to purchase the separate diary. It makes a massive difference to your chances of success.

Taking charge means taking responsibility. Responsibility for how we use and fuel our bodies. Taking responsibility sounds a bit like hard work, doesn't it? It doesn't usually feel a nice thing. People talk about shouldering responsibility and how responsibilities can weigh heavily on us.

Responsibility can be said a little differently as *response*-**ability**. The ability to respond. Taking responsibility means taking the situation you have and accepting that the responsibility is yours. I don't mean blame, I mean accepting the situation for what it is regardless of how it has come about. Some people have had their legs amputated and put on weight because they can't exercise, others have had their salad bar over the road close and a doughnut shop open in its place, some have started a family and found themselves not only chronically sleep deprived, but tidying up plates and not throwing the food away.

It doesn't matter right now how the situation arose. All that matters is that you are ready for a change. Are you?

Narcotics Anonymous had a pretty good point;

* * *

"The definition of madness is doing the same thing again and again and expecting a different result".

Taking responsibility means you taking charge, rather than letting your circumstances control you. For many people this is a little scary at first, and that's ok. Trust me. It gets better.

When you decide to take charge, good things happen as a result. It means you get to make all the decisions and that feels good. When you take charge you get to decide which direction to take. If and when obstacles crop up, you can make choices about the best way to steer around them. You can even view them as stepping-stones to take you towards your overall goals.

Are you ready for your change?

There are no shortcuts and no easy fixes. If anyone tells you there are then don't trust them. I'm sure you've discovered that easy options are short lived. I'm going to help you be long lived. Skinny Genes contains a set of strategies which are for the long term. For your entire life. I want that life to be as long and as healthy as it can be. If you want your life to be a whole lot better, this is the stuff for you.

We will start when you are ready. Are you ready to have a go? Ready to take charge? Are you ready to change yourself into the healthiest you can be?

CHAPTER THREE

How it all goes a bit wrong

The odds are stacked against us

If we understand how the body works, we can make better food choices. If we understand how it goes a bit wrong, we can do things differently. If we understand how our life is set up to make us fat, we can do something about it. This section will show you how.

Why fat is there in the first place

Fat is an energy store for lean times. Fat is vital for making some hormones and without enough of it women can't conceive. It is designed like a bank checking account you can fill up and take out of regularly. Usually that store is supposed to have only a tiny amount in it. A small positive balance. This is the healthiest way to live. Things only start to go wrong when the store is too full for too long.

Too much of a good thing

As our waistlines expand, we become less healthy.

If we are too cuddly there is more of us to carry around, which hurts our joints. Our expanding middles make it harder for us to walk, run and climb stairs. This makes us not want to be as active, which makes the problem worse. If we slow down, our metabolism slows which then burns fewer calories still.

Being bigger makes us more likely to have spots, lowers our mood and ruins the quality of our sleep. We are less likely to be able to have babies and when we do, the pregnancies are more dangerous to Mum and baby alike. As our waists expand, we increase the chance of developing diabetes and of furring up our arteries. We are more likely to die early from strokes, heart attacks and as a result of a deep vein thrombosis.

* * *

All in all, having more fat to carry around is really bad news. The really good news is that nearly all of the changes are reversible.

It is time to change direction and put all of this into reverse. You can't undo heart attacks and strokes that have happened, but you can reverse early diabetes. You can make your skin better and you can improve your sleep. You can have healthier babies and you can get your fitness back. You can improve your breathing and can improve all of your joint pains. Your mood will lift and your zest for life will turn up several notches.

We evolved

We evolved to survive. We need to eat to survive. Hunger is an inbuilt powerful biological urge to make us seek food. This carried a great survival advantage in the Stone Age.

Forty thousand years ago we didn't cook our food and had to find it ourselves. The day would have been taken up with a lot of foraging, walking to foraging places or chasing prey. Once we had our food we then needed to eat it. Eating raw plants, vegetables and meat takes a lot of chewing. This was before we learned to harness fire for cooking. The simple act of chewing could have kept us occupied nearly all day long. Only really berries, nuts, fruit and honey would have given us lots of calories for very little effort (if you discount bee stings). All of our other calories took a lot of time and effort to obtain.

Life is very different now. We have many hours a day when we aren't busy. We get more calories in a couple of mouthfuls of modern food than we might have managed all day in the Stone Age. The trouble is that our bodies and brains are set up for life in a different time.

We naturally enjoy chewing and eating constantly. It is only human to want to eat everything in front of us. We then sit and do nothing if we possibly can. All in a bid to conserve energy.

Forty thousand years ago these actions would have helped us survive and have healthy children. In the 21st century these actions kill us off early and make our children sick.

Conserving energy

Lazing around when you are not busy is a great survival strategy.

Relaxing feels good. To help our bodies lay down fat stores for the famine ahead our bodies are equipped with the urges and drives to conserve energy whenever we can.

Handily it also feels good to do stuff. Exercise releases endorphins and completing jobs and tasks gives a sense of wellbeing to encourage us to do more. Doing the things in this book will feel good too.

It is not just in modern society when people have got used to doing as little as possible. It is in our genes. Nowadays we drive when we should walk, we have ready meals when we should prepare our own food. We do everything we can to sit down and lie about because this feels good. We convince ourselves we are tired, that we need the rest and give in to our thoughts, desires and feelings to just lie on the sofa doing absolutely nothing.

If we were animals who didn't have the immediate need to go and get food, make babies or try to impress a prospective mate, then it wouldn't make sense to be wandering about or wanting to burn off lots of energy. What would be the point in that? So whenever we get the opportunity to rest, our bodies and brains are hardwired to try and take advantage of this.

We have to fight these urges. They are not helpful. We are no longer in a survival situation and our bodies will not be healthy if we don't get any exercise. I'm not outlining the powerful drives that keep us stuck to the sofa to give you an excuse. I'm simply telling you that they are quite natural.

We have to work out ways to overcome this tendency to conserve energy. When we are the wrong shape we need to do the opposite of what our bodies and minds tell us. We need to burn energy. It is time to say goodbye to the sofa a little more often.

Any excess energy is laid down

Any excess energy laid down for another day.

I have love handles. I have a bit of a belly. My bottom isn't just muscle. I have mooby man-boobs. I'm not very impressed with these. I can't imagine they impress anyone else. But this is a work in progress. It is (mostly) moving in the right direction.

I sometimes find it hard to imagine that these features of mine are the pinnacle of forty-thousand years of evolution. They are. This fat laying ability is what kept my ancestors alive in hard times. They were able to survive in conditions that I can talk about but can barely imagine. Their fat stores were life saving and this lardy layer is their gift I've inherited. I feel really lucky.

Ok, some days I don't feel all that lucky and if I'm honest I suspect I'm even a bit ungrateful. The problem is because there is no famine around the corner (probably).

One pound of fat = 3500 calories

To lose one pound of fat you need to have a five hundred calorie deficit every day for seven days in a row. If you have a 2000 day, you will need only 1500 in. Every day for a week. For one pound loss. There is a lot of energy in my fat stores.

Every ten pounds of fat I'm carrying is 35000 calories of energy. It takes two thousand calories to run a marathon. It takes about a thousand calories simply to stay alive for a day. For every ten pounds of fat in my belly, this would keep me alive and running a marathon a day for ten days in a row. With plenty of energy to spare. Without eating a single thing. I could do all of that on just water. Twenty six miles is a long way to run each day in search of food or survival. If you sit around and conserve energy and manage to even nibble a little, these fat stores will power your body for many times longer.

These fatty stores of ours are a fantastic survival feature. But they are only helpful if you have a famine to prepare for. We weren't designed to have the storage tanks full for a long period of time. Carrying around a permanent layer of survival blubber is slowly killing many of us.

Sugar cravings

We crave sugars, fats and salt. None of these are very good for us in excess. It used to be that the desire for these would have kept us alive. Now these urges are helping us into an early grave.

Sugar tastes good. Sugar tastes sweet. Sweet tastes good.

Sugar is a refined carbohydrate which delivers a quick energy hit. This lights up our brain's reward centres. The neurotransmitter dopamine is released triggering the same buzz sensation as heroin and cocaine. The same chemical is released on orgasm, on getting fantastic news such as winning the lottery and is craved by the compulsive gambler.

Sugar makes us feel good. This feel-good sensation can be addictive. There is a reason why our bodies and brains are hardwired to crave sugar and sweet stuff. This is because it gives you a lot of bang for your buck. Chewing on uncooked meat or on raw plant stems releases energy very slowly and wasn't a very efficient way of getting calories in. So it made sense that we evolved a sweet tooth.

The sugars found in fruits and in honey have been around for a very long time and this energy delivery was very efficient. It makes sense to design a system which enjoyed this taste. It would make you want to seek out more. This is exactly what happened.

Because we crave sugar like addicts, we can control this like we manage other addiction powered behaviours. We can tackle this by either gradual withdrawal and limited access to the substance you want out of your life, or by going cold-turkey and waiting for all the nasty craving sensations to go away. They eventually do. Like a lot of addictions, sugar addiction never goes away completely. The old wounds and pathways are easily re-opened. So it is best once you have kicked the habit to be aware of the risks of indulging heavily once more.

Desire for fatty foods

Food fats are very high in energy content.

Animal and plant fats add flavour to food. They have a pleasant taste which is encoded deep in our brains. This is because fat is very very high in calories. It carries even more calories than pure sugar.

It is only natural that our bodies and brains want to eat food which contains fats. If you want to control the shape of your waist you are going to want to be aware of food fat content. And probably cut it back a bit.

Fats contain some vital amines (vitamins) which are essential for healthy living but that is not an excuse. Removing dietary fat completely is simplest. Then allow yourself oily fish at least once a week. Putting a dash of olive oil on your salads is ok. Most of us sneak small amounts of fat in the diet in many other ways. But removing fats completely would be a good start if you want to make the fastest progress.

Salty pleasures

Salt makes food taste good. Too much is unpleasant. Just the right amount seems to make the food taste better. It enhances the flavour. Without it, food seems bland.

Our bodies need salt. Not much, but it is vital for health. And like all useful and vital stuff, we crave it.

We are driven to like salt in just the same way our bodies and brains are driven to seek out high calorie food, to overeat, to laze about, and to place our bodies in optimal fat laying down conditions.

Our bodies can have too much of a good thing with too much excess energy slowly killing us. It is the same with salt. Too much salt in our diet will hasten the progression towards an early grave. Through higher blood pressures and then overstraining our hearts, too much salt is bad.

Most of us have about ten times too much salt in our diets. Dial it down now. Stop adding salt to your food. Your tastebuds will adjust. You will live longer. It is worth it.

Basal metabolic rate

When we eat less and consume fewer calories, our bodies notice. This is a bit of a shame but they do.

If you eat fewer calories each day and don't pay attention, you will slow down. The basal metabolic rate slows in an effort to conserve energy. Your body thinks you might be starving. It isn't really under conscious control. This is important to realise because if you aren't aware of this you might not understand what happens.

If your body has slowed a little it will encourage you to want to sit around to try and burn fewer calories. This is ok, because this is only a signal. Just a message. Like all messages, this one can be ignored. You can stay active, you can even increase your activity levels. Your body will cope.

The point is that if you don't think about this, you might eat less, slow down, burn less, need less and then wonder why you aren't losing the inches off your waistline.

The key is to realise this will happen and be ready for it.

Stay active. Keep doing stuff. Restrict your intake but stay active. This will work.

Your body will try to alter your activity set point. Ignore it. You have energy stores to spare. Use your super-powerful brain to take charge and override the signals which will try to get your behind back in the comfy chair. You will feel the appeal. You won't want to get up - but the great thing is that once you are up and about doing stuff, the body is fine with it. It is like a grumpy teenager. It will not do anything without a severe kick up the butt. But once it is up and about it can move about perfectly well.

CHAPTER FOUR

Modern living

Abundance

We live in a life of abundance. But we are not designed to live surrounded by food. This tempts us. Most of us are able resist most things. We just can't resist temptation.

"I can resist anything but temptation."
Oscar Wilde (1854-1990), Novelist, playwright and poet.

It is very nice to have lots of stuff and to have an easy life. Unfortunately this life of comfort and plenty isn't helping us to be healthy or live longer. There are many problems which come with this luxurious life that makes efficient waist management a tricky prospect for so many of us.

We have more free time than we used to. We have labour saving devices and live in different times from only a few generations ago. Our jobs are different, we commute further and use the car far more. We have refrigeration, different shopping habits and are either too busy to cook or don't know how. We have changed the way we think about treats. We snack more than ever before. We have more calorie dense food at cheaper prices than ever. We are tempted daily by food that is specifically engineered to appeal to our tastebuds.

The odds are stacked against us. It isn't surprising that it sometimes gets a little out of control.

More free time

Modern life gives us more free time. I love my free time. My free time is what I have when I'm not at work. I love to spend time with my family, with my friends, reading books, watching films. It is great.

We are extremely fortunate to be living at a point in history in which we have more free time available than ever before. It is truly amazing how little time it takes to find, eat and digest our food. We used to spend many hours each day hunting or foraging. Chewing the food alone could have taken up most of the day. Have you ever tried to eat a raw antelope? It takes a lot of chewing.

The problem with free time is that if we aren't careful it can work against us. The same biological urges drive us, whether we are busy or have lots of free time. We will be driven to graze, to eat as much as we can and to burn as few calories as possible so we can lay down fat. It is crucial to think about your free time and the way you spend it. Is it helping your quest for a beach-ready body? Or is it working against you? Eating and sitting around not burning calories is the default setting. This is what we need to address.

Practically this means you shouldn't have snacks available when you are resting on the sofa. You should deliberately be doing stuff that burns calories during your free time. This energy burning movement will keep your body healthy. We were not designed to sit around too long. After a few days rest we would have been foraging or off to join the hunt. We weren't designed to be sedentary for weeks, months and years at a time.

Keeping busy naturally curbs our hunger. Use this fact. When we are out walking or running in the countryside we don't snack nearly as much. For the moment I will ignore the recent trend of taking on board energy drinks and snacks while working out - this is stupid, unnecessary and the result of misleading advertising. You don't need to eat to exercise. You can read more about that in my book '*Beginner's Guide to Running*'. I will stop ranting now.

Labour saving devices

I have a lot of gadgets. I am very lucky. I have a car which takes me to work. I have a bicycle which is also very efficient (but not as warm, safe or dry). I have a washing machine to clean my clothes. If I pay for the extra electricity, the same device even dries them for me. I have a chainsaw which chops through wood with no effort on my part. I have a lot of toys.

I don't need any of them. But they are very nice. I have to spend very little energy on my day to day tasks. When I want food to eat I can either pay for someone else to give me food or prepare it myself. If I pay someone else in a restaurant or take-out it is even hot and ready to eat. I can microwave packaged meals giving me ready to eat food in only a couple of minutes. Even if I buy my own meat and vegetables, I have very sharp knives and an oven which will cook the food, making it easy for me to chew and digest.

* * *

Before we had ovens and fire we would have had raw meat to eat. Raw vegetables and raw everything. These sorts of foods take a lot of chewing to get all of the nutrients out. No wonder we came to like fruit and honey. Eating fruit, berries, nuts and seeds must have seemed wonderfully easy compared to raw root vegetables and meat.

The disadvantage of the labour saving gadgets and the lifestyle I enjoy is that I am able to be very lazy. I can pamper my inner sloth. I hardly burn any energy in food preparation, in keeping my house nice, in heating my home and keeping it safe. This means that my waistline expands if I don't watch out. I have to think about spending more of my free time in burning the calories that my ancestors would have burned simply by staying alive.

It is funny really how much we've evolved. We've developed so much and saved so much energy that to stay healthy we have to go out and deliberately burn calories. The same calories we've saved by making our lives more efficient.

Jobs

The jobs that many of us do have changed beyond all recognition from only a few hundred years ago.

Going back thousands of years, we would have worked together in small groups moving from camp to camp working the bushes and grasslands to find the best pickings of berries, nuts, fruit and the easiest animals to catch. When we had used up all the local resources and had to move progressively further to gather food, we would simply move on. We moved on to the next suitable area.

When we started to farm we settled in one place. Here we would have worked the land and tended our animals from dawn to dusk for all the months of the year the weather was favourable. When the weather became more hostile we would have sat around to conserve energy, trying to make our food stores last until the next season's crop became available.

There would have been no snacking.

After the industrial revolution, jobs changed. A few rich people did very well out of it, the rest of us would have been the workers. If we were lucky enough to have jobs. The work was hard and the hours very long. There were few breaks and the wages low. There simply wasn't the money to buy more food than you needed.

Again, there was very little snacking.

Only during the last fifty years have things started to change significantly. The motor car, the jet engine, the telephone, the computer, fridges, plastics, pesticides and efficient farming techniques have happened. Food abounds in the Western world more than at any point in history. The proportion of the population at risk of actual starvation is now extremely small.

More people die in the West from too much food than from too little.

The problem these days is there is too much food available. Most of us even get to eat at work. We eat at meal times, we munch on our breaks. We nibble on the way to work and on the way home again. Many of us even graze during the working day. Our purses contain chocolate and sweets, our desk drawers have snacks - just for emergencies. We have take-outs, sugar in our drinks, cream in our coffees and scoff muffins, doughnuts, bagels and cake frequently throughout the week. These are extra calories in. More calories than we maybe need.

* * *

How often at work is it someone's birthday and they bring in cake? How often do reps bring sweet treats for the office staff? How often has someone been on holiday and brings back some tasty souvenir for their colleagues? If it is Friday, does someone go to the cake shop? Do people fetch edible treats just because work is busy and we all deserve a little boost?

It is easily done. Our jobs have changed. They have changed beyond all recognition. They are nice. I'm very happy with what I do. But there are more opportunities than ever to put calories in while burning fewer and fewer.

Commute

We used to forage and hunt near where we slept. When the journey to fetch food and water became too great, we moved on. We moved our tribe to a better area.

When we became farmers we would live on or near the land we tended. We would live near or among our livestock. Commuting was a foreign concept. When we started to work in factories we started to journey to work. Most of us would live in cheap housing near the local factory. We lived near our work. We wouldn't come home for lunch as the extended lunchtime break was hundreds of years away. The lunch hour was not yet invented.

As the last century ticked by, more of us became able to afford houses away from the crowded conditions near the factories. We moved out of the centre of towns and the suburban life began. This meant travelling further to our places of work. The motor car and improved public transport let us make this journey easily. The daily commute is now a feature of working life for many or most of us.

This commute is generally done while seated. Cars, buses, boats, horses - they all involve sitting down. Bicycles are sitting down too, but at least they burn a few more calories. Our jobs are sat down mostly. Our commute to work is often sitting. Our breaks and meal times are seated, along with our journey home.

To make things worse, a lot of us announce once home;

'Wow, I'm so tired, I really need a sit down'.

We then sit at the table or on the sofa to eat our supper. We sit in our beds and then sleep. Repeating the whole process the next day.

It is hardly any wonder that we don't burn very many calories each day. It is hardly any wonder we often manage to eat more than we burn off. It is not really a surprise that society at large is gradually increasing in size.

What surprises me is the situation isn't worse than it is. This is a testament to many people's effort and will power. However this is other people. It isn't you and me. What matters to us is our waistline. We want to look good naked in front of the mirror. We want our joints to stop hurting and to be able to climb stairs without a serious medical risk each time.

Fridges

Our refrigerators make life easy. We only need to go shopping once a week. We could go out even less than that. I know people who have their weekly or monthly shop delivered to their home. This is convenient but super lazy. It will not help you much in your quest for a sexier body. The only way it can help is that you might be less tempted by the junk food in the shop.

Convenient shopping doesn't encourage you to buy fresh produce. It doesn't get you off the sofa and moving around the shops. You don't get the exercise benefit of pushing a trolley. You don't get the benefit of carrying shopping bags and getting a weights workout.

We no longer milk our own cows. We no longer dig, sow, plant, tend and harvest our own vegetables. We expend very few calories in getting food onto our plates.

Our fridges are becoming larger. We fill them up with more and more junk. We have oven chips and not frozen vegetables filling our freezers. We have drawers full of ice cream. We have ever more alcohol crammed into our fridges. We often choose to keep high calorie juices and cream there. We rarely use them for chilled water. Even with a slice of fresh lemon.

Shopping habits

Our shopping habits give us opportunities to buy in bulk. If we buy in bulk there is often food around the house. Often high calorie food which is easier to eat than to prepare a fresh meal with lots of healthy vegetables.

We buy salad items, but they go over and we end up throwing them away. It is easier to reach for the cookie jar than it is to make a salad. We are all naturally lazy. It isn't our fault, but when you are tired it is easy to make poor choices.

We are seduced in the supermarket by the offers. We buy the stuff that is put on the ends of aisles. We buy things with attractive packaging. This is how supermarkets make their money. They understand our psychology. The food manufacturers don't have your best interests at heart. They simply want profit. Food producers make their wares attractive. Easy to prepare with no effort on your part. They add lots of sugar and fat, with plenty of salt too. This is because it seduces us. This food appeals to our tastebuds.

It isn't complex to understand - but these are poor food choices. Stuff you have to put together and make yourself is going to be better for you. Taking time and effort to prepare food burns more calories and gives you more control over what you are putting in the top end. This is a good place to begin. There is a lot more effort required in terms of making sensible choices, but it is at least a start.

It is time to stop being seduced by the offers. Stop listening to the shouting of the packaging. Improve your shopping choices. There are no other sensible options. It is more tricky to be disciplined with your eating if your cupboards and refrigerator are crammed with unhelpful stuff. It is like entering a duel with one hand tied behind your back. With a hat pulled over your eyes. With your ankles bound. It is not just going to end well if you start like this.

Cooking abilities

Your ability to cook can help or hinder you.

If you cannot prepare food very well, you are not alone. If you can, then you have fewer excuses not to eat well. Modern living doesn't lead us to want to cook. We have more disposable income than ever before. Many of us can afford to eat out occasionally. Many of us can eat take-outs. Even once a month is a lot from a health point of view.

A hundred years ago we would have eaten out perhaps never, but no more than a couple of times a year for anyone but the seriously rich. Ordinary people like us just wouldn't have done this. We would have prepared and eaten our own food. We would have used the leftovers and would have bought and used whichever ingredients were cheapest. Affording only seasonal produce. Exotic fruits and dishes from all around the world wouldn't have been an option even only a generation ago.

This has all changed. Our corner shops are filled with TV-dinners, ready meals and foods from around the world. You can pretty much get anything you want, from anywhere on the planet, all year around. This hasn't encouraged our creative skills. It is easier now to eat out than to learn how to cook a particular type of cuisine. Because we have more free time and a lower inclination to use it for food preparation, our skills have diminished. This burns fewer calories and encourages us to eat larger portions than is really very good for us.

Car use

Our car use has increased. This isn't really news. The motor car has gone from dangerous plaything of the rich and famous to a dangerous everyday gadget of nearly everyone. Many households have one for each adult. Even our teenagers at high schools and university own cars.

Cars are really handy. I love having a car. I can carry lots of stuff easily. I stay warm and dry. I can choose my own music. I don't have to make small-talk with strangers. I don't have to wait in the rain for it to arrive. I don't even have to walk very far to get in it.

It is not good for my health or my waistline. I would miss it very much if I didn't have it and it provides a lot of convenience. And this is precisely the point.

We have collectively become very dependant on cars. We don't walk very far each day. Few of us run or cycle anywhere. We use the car for very short journeys and this doesn't help our curvey middles. Our health suffers because of the car. Yours. Mine. Nearly everybody's.

Perception of treats

When I was a child I was very lucky. My parents loved me and wanted me to be happy. They would from time to time buy me treats. These would be perhaps sweets, maybe an iced lolly or an ice cream on holiday.

My grandparents used to do the same. I was a conniving little brat, going out of my way to try and persuade them to give me more. I'm not very proud of that now. Though I suspect this behaviour was not unique.

I didn't have treats every week when I was young. As the years went by they increased in frequency (which was nice). When I started to get pocket-money I would buy treats for myself as often as I could. I wasn't really a child who saved much. Instant gratification was more my style.

The problem with this approach is it taught me sweet stuff was what you obtained at every opportunity. When I became older and went to university I did much the same with beer and junk food. Spend all your money, get lots of nice stuff and enjoy the moment. Think about the consequences later. Maybe.

This wasn't very good for my overall health or waistline. It didn't even make me very happy. It certainly cost all my money and started a spiral of debt that has made the subsequent years much harder than they needed to be.

When we get into the habit of treating ourselves daily, this can be a hard one to shake. Treating and rewarding ourselves with foody things is widespread but not very helpful. Many of us have taken to having treats every day. They have lost their childhood power and the impact of rarity. They are now commonplace. Many of my patients reward themselves with a small chocolate bar each day. As it is only a small one, they can justify this to themselves. Having sweet puddings or deserts are another way to reward yourself. These are a daily habit for many.

In many ways having small frequent treats is lovely, it is nice to be in a position to be able to do this. When you fill up your car, there are treats at the counter. Why not have one? Or more? I'm not saying we should deprive ourselves, but I am saying we should think about how often we actually do this. If you are serious about managing you waist, then the treats may warrant a rethink.

Dr Phil Harley

50/50 poison

There is poisonous food about. This is the 50/50 food. You might not have heard of it but it is very dangerous.

Fifty-fifty foods are poisonous because if you eat them your health will suffer. Eat enough of them and they will kill you. That is the definition of poison. The trouble is that like all the best poisons from childhood fairy tales, they are very tempting. They make you want to eat them.

Fifty percent carbohydrate and fifty percent fat is the ratio of the 50/50 foods. Half sugar and half fat. No protein, no vitamins, no fibre. The problem with this food is that is tastes so good. It floods our brain with happy chemicals, making us want more and more and more.

Food with the evil magic formula is not hard to find.

* * *

These are usually the foods we reward ourselves with. They are comfort foods and will slowly poison us to death. We are often willing victims. These include foods most of us love to eat; … doughnuts, carrot cake, chocolate cake, cream cakes, chocolate eclairs, cookies, shortbread, flapjack, chocolate, custard and Twinkies.

They are everywhere and we are easily seduced. Be aware.

Faulty off switch

When we eat foods with the fifty-fifty mix of sugars and fats we feel good.

Dopamine is released in our brains giving us a hit. These highs are addictive. We crave them. This dopamine surge is something we will actively seek out. It hits the pleasure centres of our brains and the reward centres.

Fifty-fifty foods are chock full of calories.

These empty calories are not at all good for you. They are not going to contribute towards your quest for a better looking figure. Your naked appearance is probably not going to be enhanced very much.

They have nothing about them which is good. They have no

vitamins and no fibre. Alarmingly they also seem to produce no stop-signal. For some reason, our bodies don't really put the brakes on while chomping away. We can't really tell very well when we've had enough. We simply keep eating.

We get huge numbers of calories in before even drawing breath. Because they don't require much chewing we shovel them in at speed. Because there is so little fibre and bulk it passes easily through our stomach and into our gut for digesting. The chemical make up means our stomach empties rapidly and we can keep putting food in the top end without becoming full.

It is very very easy to overeat with the fifty-fifty foods. You can eat your entire day's calorie allowance in about three minutes. Maybe quicker if you work at it. Afterwards you may feel a little sick. You may feel a little remorse to go with the nausea. It is too late. The calories are in.

Massive action is required if we are not to allow ourselves to become poisoned.

There isn't really an antidote. We need to be aware of the poisoning risks. Every day we should be on the lookout for foods which might do this to us. We should be aware and beware of stuff we desire and which we might want to shove down our throats a bit too fast. Too quickly to hear the full signal when it eventually emerges. We should avoid situations where we see this stuff. We shouldn't buy it. We should politely turn it down when it is offered.

It isn't easy to avoid this stuff. It is everywhere. And it really does taste good. I do know. But in our quest, we will have to be better. We will have to somehow turn aside and stay strong.

Opportunistic snacking

When we have the opportunity to eat, we tend to. We pick at whatever food is around. Even if we aren't hungry.

It is remarkable how much we can put in our mouth when we are so full that it even hurts a little. This is opportunistic snacking.

Basically, if it is there we will eat it. If we see it we want it. This is the snacking version of the seafood diet joke (*I'm on a seafood diet.* Really? *Yes, when I see food, I eat it*). Only it isn't a joke. This is a see-food snack issue. Animals have a word for this - grazing. We humans feel the need to graze because our stomachs never know when we will next eat again, so we are compelled to try and eat everything in sight. We don't really have a very good off switch. It is not just you. It is you, me and everybody. Some people's off switches are a bit better than others. For most of us if it is there we will eat it.

There have been scientific studies on this. On seeing food and wanting it. It doesn't really seem to matter what it is, if it is there we will eat it. It is not really a matter of willpower. The mind over matter thing worked for only so long and then the subjects studied simply gave in. If they were tired, stressed or distracted, they gave in more quickly.

What can you do about this? Hide the food. Put the snacks away where you can't see them. If you are in the habit of wandering around your kitchen when you are a bit bored, hungry, lonely or sad then put them in cupboards. If you tend to open the cupboards to see if there is food to be had, then hide them at the back where your eyes don't see them. I'm aware that your brain will be able to find them if it wants, but keeping out of that initial sightline is a vital first step.

Some of us need a bit more help in the first few weeks and months. Some of us need to have no snack food anywhere in the cupboards, nothing in the house, nor in the garage, carport or nearby outbuildings. We need to have no cash in the drawer, wallet, purse or car to be able to dash out and purchase high calorie snacks in a moment of weakness.

Talking of moments of weakness. That drive-by cruising of the refrigerator and opening of cupboards and drawers hoping to find a forgotten snack or piece of chocolate isn't a good habit. It needs to stop. It does you no favours and no good will come of it. When you feel the urge to do that, wait for it to pass. Urges come in waves. Wait for the wave to subside. The getting up out of the chair is good, but the direction needs to be away from the foody areas.

Walk around for the same five minutes until the feeling passes. Burn twenty calories here, don't put any extra in. The urge will fade. It always does.

CHAPTER FIVE

Eating patterns

Emotional eating

Eating to fill an emotional hole doesn't work very well.

It is a fact that emotional holes are not best filled by food.

The hole is essentially bottomless. There is no amount of food that can be put in which will fill the void. Eating will temporarily make some people feel better. They eat stuff that gives them comfort feelings. This is due to dopamine release in the brain. The food we eat when young becomes associated with safe and happy feelings. These can be triggered by comfort eating. The problem arises because the underlying sad feelings or the loneliness will still be there when the dopamine surge wears off. Sometimes only minutes later.

It is very easy for some people to get in the habit of a comfort eating cycle.

* * *

Feel sad, want to distract yourself, eat snack, feel better, snack wears off, still feel sad, eat another snack ...

Becoming aware of this possible behaviour pattern around food is half the battle. This is a good thing. The rest of the battle is changing one's life, or the way one looks at life to steer clear of the initial sad feeling.

When we feel sad this is a feeling that we have to generate in our own heads. It isn't there before we choose to think of it. You can change this.

If we are feeling sad or lonely, unappreciated and isolated we need to correct this emotion. Food is not the best way to do this. Connecting with others is. If it is not practical to do this in person, do this in the comfort of your own imagination. Take a minute or two to consider how much you are loved. Someone who dotes on you. Unconditionally. Your Mom, your spouse, your pet. They all count.

Whether you choose to do this in person, over the telephone or internet doesn't matter. Whether you choose to connect by talking, texting, emailing, sending photos or by meeting up doesn't matter too much either. It also doesn't seem to make a huge amount of difference if you actually do it or if you simply think about someone close to you. It does work better if you reach out and tell someone how much they mean to you, but it can be effective if you simply consider how important they are in your life.

All of this makes your brain feel better and will help your mood more than any high calorie comfort food. Connecting with others is a good daily habit to cultivate.

Snacking habits

Snacking is unhelpful. This is eating between meals and usually isn't at all necessary. Many of us have habits that fill our faces with food. These habits include:

- *Absent minded snacks.*
- *Procrastinating by feeding.*
- *Eating out of habit.*
- *Social munching.*
- *Drunken grazing.*
- *Fear of hypoglycaemia (low blood sugar) and panic eating.*

When we are not concentrating, we will tend to put anything within reach into our mouths. While surfing the net, while watching a film, while driving in heavy traffic. It is easy to do. It is time to stop this. If you don't think about the food, you are probably not enjoying it all that much or tasting it. Notice when you do this and pay more attention. Do you *really* want that snack? Really?

We put off stuff we don't want to do. We do this for a whole range of reasons. We call this procrastinating. We procrastinate by texting friends, checking our emails, going shopping or tidying up. We do all sorts of things apart from the task at hand. We also eat. We tend to eat junk when we procrastinate. It would be better for your day and your waistline if you simply got on with whatever you are putting off.

Eating at certain times of day is partly because our days work well with some structure, but partly habit. Snacking on certain things at particular times can become habit too. Eat when you are hungry. Not just because it is time to eat. You are not a robot. You have free will. Use it.

Social snacking. When we are in the company of others and food is shared, we eat it. We don't want to seem ungrateful. Even if we don't want it or are not even very hungry. Learn to politely decline it. Don't offer stuff to others and put them in this situation. Be nice by all means - but not always with high calorie food options.

When we have some alcohol in our systems we tend to want to eat. We either graze on bar snacks, eat large meals, eat take-out on the way home, or fix ourselves a little something when we get there. We don't make good decisions when drunk and food is no exception. We often don't need the calories we eat while drunk, we don't hear the full signal and generally make poor choices. Alcohol itself is high in calories and we frequently mix it with other drinks that contain even more. This is often in the evening after we have finished our food for the day. These are all bonus calories.

The last snacking pattern I want to mention is low blood sugar. Unless you are on medications to treat your diabetes, there is no need to fear low blood sugar. We have got very used to never feeling the slightest bit hungry. Being hungry isn't bad for you. There is no need to reach for calories if you feel faint headed. Nothing bad will happen. Most of us have got used to completely the wrong sensations and we then reach for food to prevent some terrible imagined tragedy. The real tragedy is that nothing bad would happen and we simply put in way more calories than we actually need. Even in a life or death situation, one hundred calories is all you need. Less than half a Snickers.

Changing old habits

Changing habits feels weird at first.

Changing your snacking and eating habits will change your waistline. If you change them, you can do better. If you do not, you are not likely to make much of a difference. But it is not always easy. It feels strange when you change old habits. We are used to them. Like a comfortable pair of shoes. But even the comfiest shoes need replacing. Do not panic. Doing things differently takes time. It takes a while to do stuff better and even more for it to feel natural.

Think of it like brushing your teeth. For most of us this feels pretty natural. We do it at the same time each day, in the same way and with the same hand. If I asked you to use the other hand and do it four times a day you'd struggle initially. My patients who've had a hand in plaster and had to switch hands are able to achieve something on day one. They are pretty adept by the end of week two and it feels natural by the time the cast is removed in six to eight weeks.

Much the same is true about changing your eating schedule and habits. Do-able with a deal of effort on day one, but not very good. Much better by the end of the first fortnight and by the time we get to eight weeks it feels much more natural. We are creatures of habit and handily we have the capacity to deliberately teach ourselves new habits. The outcome is well worth the effort when you able to effortlessly eat well, aren't hungry, feel more happy, healthier, fitter, thinner, become more toned, have more energy and look noticeably better naked.

The brain doesn't take long to train to learn a new trick, but to make it automatic takes effort. This is because the inside of the brain actually changes shape. It does this by strengthening the connections along the nerve pathways. It literally changes as you do new things. That is why it feels easier with time. After consistent careful practice the changes can last a lifetime.

International sports stars snack less than me. They enjoy it as much I'm sure, but have got out of the habit of grazing like I do. They simply don't think about it as often. We too can do this with a bit of effort and application. It doesn't much to get started. It gets progressively easier. Habits take a few weeks to ingrain. The precise number of days will vary between people and in different situations. The research scientists tell us it is about sixty days for most of us. Learning new stuff is much quicker than ingraining an automatic behaviour and can set you on the right path immediately.

> *Learning can be really rapid. You can change the habit of a lifetime after reading it once.*

Think about the way you drive to work. If you take half an hour through town and always sit in the same traffic queue at the same place, you might be pretty used to that journey. If I showed you a shortcut or turnpike which enabled you take to ten minutes off your commute each and every time, you might not need showing twice.

Some things in this book are like being shown a new shortcut. After a while the old route will become overgrown. You could still go that way but probably will choose not to.

CHAPTER SIX

How to reverse the trend

Making better choices

Changing your approach to all things food and movement related is clearly a big ask. This is made easier by breaking it down into manageable chunks. Do lots of different small things. Do them better. Work on them bit by bit, do them better and better in your daily quest towards your target goals.

It is all about making better choices.

We live our lives making thousands of choices each and every day. What to wear, which way to walk, what to say, when to go to the bathroom. We get to choose what we eat, when we eat and how many bites to take. The choices we make each and every day make us who we are. We live and die by the choices we make. They affect everything we do.

Free will is great. But it comes at a price.

* * *

Every thing we do has consequences. All the choices you make each and every day have knock-on effects. Sometimes the effect is large and immediate. For example, when not to cross a busy street. Sometimes the choices will take decades to have a noticeable effect. For example, whether to smoke a cigarette.

Making better choices each and every day around food will produce the results you want. They don't have to be huge or difficult choices. But you will need to make a lot of them. The more of these that become automatic, the better. If you consistently make good food choices without thinking, then when you are in a stressful situation or distracted you are likely to make an improved selection.

In addiction medicine there is an acronym to describe when people are more likely to make poor choices. Poor in terms of their long term health and wellbeing. This is when people are **Hungry**, **A**lone, **L**onely or **T**ired (HALT). Its origins are from Alcoholics Anonymous but it is helpful for us all, highlighting situations where we are at risk of poor choices.

Getting new habits is about making these new and better choices consistently. It is the consistency which will produce the best results.

> *Your future depends on your actions today. Everything you do has consequences.*

It is time to invest in your future. It is time to start doing stuff today which will give you a better life in years to come. Managing your waistline the Skinny Genes way is a great way to start. While you are motivated you can start making actions. Start completing the diary today. The one at the back of this book. If you have the e-book version, buy the separate diary, it's worth the effort.

Acting against your nature

Habits are a vital evolutionary adaptation to save space. Brain function takes up a lot of energy. Twenty percent of our daily intake is used to power the little grey cells. When you are in a survival situation every little counts. Any strategy that used less brain computing power would be advantageous. That is why we have habits.

Habits are automated pieces of behaviour which require no conscious thought and run on autopilot. As much as sixty per cent of your daily activities are habit driven.

Habits can be brief or long, simple or complex. They may be physical, mental or emotional.

They all follow the same pattern of cue, behaviour and a reward. They can be interrupted and disrupted relatively easily. The trick is to spot them and decide what to adjust. Changing them involves doing the new thing for about sixty days consistently.

Once a new one is learned it takes over. They are never completely unlearned, so watch out for the old triggers. *Just when you thought it was safe to go back ...*

Once learned they take charge of unconscious behaviour, which is their whole point. Even if it is harmful or goes against common sense. So an unhealthy habit persists even if you should know better.

Choose your habits wisely.

Calorie counting

Skinny Genes is all about showing how to make better food choices. It is about accepting that our nature will make us eat poorly if given half the chance.

Making better choices means eating less and moving more.

We should pick nutritious food options. We should not eat too much at any one sitting. We should do a lot of things that we don't always get around to. To get the right calorie balance each day, counting the calories in and the calories out is _really really_ helpful.

When you first do this it may seem like hard work and a faff. It gets easier. You soon learn to guess calories accurately. Most of us underestimate portion sizes to begin with.

I get my patients to pour into a bowl what they think a helping of cereal looks like. They often pour between two and four times the recommended serving. This exercise produces similar results with pasta. Butter and spreads are not very well guessed either.

There are lots of applications and programs which you can use to help you count calories. It is important not to overestimate what you burn. The amount you burn each day is your basal metabolic rate (background energy need) added together with your output for the day (work, rest and play).

Some apps calculate only the energy spent during exercise and some include your basal metabolic rate. While the precise numbers don't matter too much, if you end up not losing what you hope to, then think about why this might be. If you overestimate your output you may allow yourself too many treats and be surprised when the waist isn't being managed as well as you expect from your sums.

Getting started

Making changes feels a little strange at first. Like a new pair of shoes. You are not alone in this feeling. Saying **no** to snacks and having smaller portions may also feel tricky initially.

Your brain will give you hunger and panic signals when you start putting less in. It is sending you misleading information out of habit and not *actual* need. The thermostat needs adjusting down. The signals and feedback will become quieter over time.

How you start will depend on what else is going on in your life. How busy you are, how motivated and how much exercise you have started doing.

While it possible to do everything on day one, it will give you less of a shock factor if you approach this gradually.

* * *

On day one perhaps park in the furthest parking space, not the closest. Leave a forkful of food on each plate. You might eat a little slower. Try a glass of water before lunch and perhaps a little less alcohol at the end of the day.

This will help. All of it. Little by little you will see what is achievable. The most important thing on day one is to think about what you are doing.

Think about what you are eating, what drinks you have and how much you *really* do in terms of exercise. It makes a massive difference if you write it down. Everything. Be honest. Don't worry if it seems challenging. It gets better.

CHAPTER SEVEN

Learn from our ancestors

Lessons from the past

Our ancestors did very well. They survived, they replicated. They produced you. Eventually.

The diets and lifestyle of those we evolved from clearly got some things right. We survived. As a species, being overweight wasn't really the challenge we face today. Why not? What was different? What did we used to do that we no longer do? How differently did we eat?

We can never know for sure, but archaeological anthropologists think we used to eat food very different to today's. There was no modern wheat, there were no refined sugars. Cereals and oats were absent. For a lot of our life on the planet we didn't even cook our food. There would have been no potatoes, no rice, no pasta and very few eggs.

* * *

To chew raw food takes a lot of time and calories. Gathering or hunting food takes a lot of energy and we would have remained active throughout our lives. When we were older we couldn't afford to slow down but would have played an active role in tending the camp and looking after the younger members of the tribe.

What can we learn from this? We should stay as active as possible. We should try not to have excess food in our diet. If we do, then burn off these extra calories before too long. We should keep up the roughage in our diet and eat as varied an intake as possible. Hunter-gatherer societies ate a much more varied diet than we now achieve. Also, for many of us our digestive systems do not handle wheat or milk proteins very well.

To keep from being hungry we should keep busy and eat more slowly.

Controlling hunger

The four very best ways to control hunger pangs:

- *Be busy*
- *Exercise hard*
- *Have a full belly*
- *Ignore it*

When you are busy or exercising hard you tend to have less hunger. When you are sat still with nothing much to occupy you, the hunger returns unless you have a full stomach.

Controlling hunger by simply ignoring it can work well too - more on this later.

Keeping your mind occupied will mean the hunger signal becomes quieter. This makes sense because if you are already busy doing something, this may have been finding or preparing food. It could also have been if you were evading danger or making or looking after babies and children. It makes no sense for your body to be hungry in those situations. So you aren't nowadays when your body is in similar situations.

If you are chasing a rabbit, rat or antelope you will need to keep your mind on the task. If you are running five miles to find the nearest beehive with its reward of golden honey you will need to be focused on the job in hand. If you are running away from a lion you will need to be just doing running. Thinking about food won't help you here. The hunger signal appropriately turns down in volume when you are doing these things.

The hunger signal also turns down a few notches when you are full. This makes sense because having your stomach explode wouldn't be helpful. When your stomach feels full, stretched, bloated or distended, you feel less hungry and usually slow down the rate at which you put food into your mouth.

So to feel less hungry; you should keep busy, move more or have a fuller feeling tummy.

Distraction

Being busy distracts you from eating.

While you are doing something else, then the mouth isn't being filled with food for as many minutes as you are busy. There are only twenty four lots of sixty minutes in a day. The more of these you are not eating, the better.

Distracting yourself can offset your hunger. Managing when you choose to eat is easier when you are busy. We all have different lives and the way we each busy ourselves will be different.

The more you practice delaying the time at which you eat, the easier it becomes. Your body learns over time to adjust the signals it gives you, driving you to seek food. They become quieter.

Like all habit change, this takes a few weeks and months to get properly used to. This sounds a long time away on day one, but you will find as each day and week pass you find it easier to put-off the time when you eat.

Hunger is a signal

Hunger is a biological urge. It drives you to action. It impels your body to go and find food.

This urge for food when our stomachs are empty is a survival thing. If we didn't desire food, we might spend too much time doing other stuff and simply run out of fuel. An animal or early human without this drive would not have survived very long.

It makes perfect sense that the desire to eat constantly whenever the opportunity arises is inbuilt and powerful.

All of our inbuilt powerful desires carry a survival advantage. Desire to drink when we are thirsty is the most obvious similar one.

The urges to purge waste products so they don't accumulate are good examples. Powerful biological urges drive us to seek out healthy mates, impress them and want to have sex with them. This helped us pass on our genes. We have drives which make us want to keep our offspring safe and we have jealousy which makes us want to keep our mates for ourselves to protect our genetic interests. We are driven to seek gossip as this is a rich source of information which can potentially help us in our groups. Vital insider information to assist us in our pursuit of status, mate selection and choosing which friends to trust. Or not.

Hunger is just one of these many survival signals. It is natural, but just like some of the other signals we don't have to follow it all of the time.

You will not die

Hunger isn't fatal.

You will not die if you feel hungry. This sounds exaggerated and overdramatic. But is an important point. Hunger is only a signal. It is only a message. It is part of your body or unconscious brain telling your conscious brain something. It is an urge and nothing more. We don't always follow all of our urges all of the time. At least I hope you don't.

If I followed all my urges, my life would be a little different. They are not always socially appropriate. Your urges may be perfectly acceptable and ok to follow in polite company. But I suspect you might be like me and want to exercise a little control. Not all the time, but sometimes.

Hunger is just an urge. A signal, nothing more. You can choose to listen and act on it …or you can simply notice it. Then carry on with whatever you were doing.

The urge to sleep, wee, poop, the sex urge and the urge to bop someone on the nose are just some of the urges I suppress from time to time, along with the hunger urge. You will have your own urges to suppress. You and I are only human after all. Hunger is just one more of these.

Learn to listen to it, thank it for sharing and then to get on with what you are doing. You will gain a little control over something that many of my patients feel controls them. This can be extremely liberating.

CHAPTER EIGHT

Manage hunger

Eat more slowly

Eating more slowly helps you to feel full sooner. Stretching the stomach walls sends a full signal. Full signals are also triggered by food content. Your stomach wall has chemical receptors which detect protein and fats, sending you a full signal. It is not just how much and how fast the food arrives in the stomach. Carbohydrates and the 50:50 mix don't seem to trigger the full signal very well. These foods which are dangerous. We risk overeating as the normal signals are not triggered.

Your stomach has stretch detectors embedded in the walls. When the stomach is stretched, these nerves fire. They send signals to the brain via the nerves and by chemicals released into the bloodstream. This signal says:

"Stop eating, you are full now."

* * *

The brain hears this and you slow or stop your eating. When you aren't listening to this signal, you can keep on eating leading to painful over-stretching of the stomach and taking on more calories than you really need in that sitting.

You can use this full signal to help guide your eating. This takes a bit of doing at first if you aren't used to listening out for the signal. If you put the brakes on and pause between mouthfuls you will hear the full signal a little earlier.

My mother used to tell me it takes twenty minutes for your tummy to tell you when you are full. She isn't a doctor. Twenty years of medicine later, I've learned she was pretty much right all along. Eat a meal slowly over twenty minutes, or give yourself a twenty minute pause and you will allow your tummy to send you any full signals. If you are still hungry at that point - eat a little more.

Glycaemic index

Carbohydrates are absorbed more quickly than any other food component. They make your blood sugar rise. This gives a brief energy boost and feel-good buzz.

This can become addictive as many of us are only too aware. We aren't really designed to run high blood sugars, so our pancreas releases a little protein called insulin when the blood sugar level rises. Insulin brings down the sugar and does so pretty well. It causes sugar to be taken up into cells for instant use, with any excess converted to fat stores.

The overall effect is that sugary foods cause a brief rise in blood sugar but your body acts to bring it right back down again. Lots of my patients report a tired, washed out feeling caused by this rapid rise and fall of blood sugar. The repeated highs and so-called '*sugar lows*' can feel exhausting.

* * *

Eating carbohydrates with fibre slows down the release of sugars. Some carbohydrates (the complex or long chained ones) release their energy more slowly. Some doctors think that if your body is used to having slow release energy, that this helps stop you developing diabetes. Foods that release their energy slowly have a low glycaemic index (GI).

The glycaemic index is a measure of how fast your body gets the energy compared to glucose. Sugar, cornflakes, fruit juice, bread and potatoes have a high GI.

High GI = bad. Low GI = good.

Brown bread has an even higher GI than white bread, so don't assume it is the healthy option. It simply doesn't contain enough fibre to slow down the sugar release.

Honey, *Mars* bars and chocolate are lower GI than bread, pasta or potatoes. Some whole fruit is lower because of its fibre. Peas, beans and lentils are lower than that. Vegetables, seeds and nuts are lower still. Thinking about how high or low the GI score of your food can help you control how much your body releases the insulin which fills up your adipocytes (fat cells).

Basic food components

The three food components that affect hunger are **protein**, **fat** and **carbohydrate**.

Protein fills you up and most people should probably eat more.

Fat makes you feel full. Even though it has lots of calories, it can be kept in a lot of meals. It adds flavour and a pleasant texture. Some fats are better for you than others.

Carbohydrates (carbs) are simply energy. Nothing more. Most of us need to eat a lot less carbohydrate.

Protein is found in vegetables in large quantities. In meat, fish and poultry too. Beans, nuts, milk and eggs all have plenty of protein. This protein content will help you feel full and stay fuller longer. Proteins form the building blocks of muscle. If we are controlling our waist and losing a bit of weight, we will need plenty of protein in our diet to help keep our muscles the way they are and not have them waste away as our middle starts to shrink.

The best way to get enough protein is to eat lots and lots of vegetables. A rule of thumb I use with my patients is to ask them to quadruple their intake. I ask them to go away and times it by four. That usually does the trick.

Fat is high in calories. It is the most calorie dense food. You should use fat carefully. With fatty foods it is very easy to eat your entire daily allowance in one sitting.

It used to be thought that furring up of our arteries was directly related to the amount of fat in the diet. This is no longer thought to be the case. It is a lot more complex than that. Being overweight is worse for your arteries than the amount of fat you eat. Having a large middle is just as bad for your health as smoking.

Some patients worry about their cholesterol levels. Being too round puts these up along with your genetic make up. The amount of fat on your plate doesn't really match up very well at all with fats in the bloodstream. We now learn that cholesterol levels themselves aren't very well linked to who gets a heart attack. We know cholesterol lowering medicines help with heart attack prevention, but they probably work by decreasing inflammation in arterial walls rather than lowering actual cholesterol levels.

What does this mean for you? It means if you would like, you can have fat in your meal because it tastes nice. Just be careful how much you put in.

It probably matters a bit which type of fats your choose. This is partly to do with the omega 3 content (humans don't extract this well from plant based sources but do from fish oils), this stuff seems to be cardio-protective. The best source of omega rich healthy oils are oily fish. Tinned tuna doesn't count. The best are sardines, herring, sprats and mackerel. Trout and salmon are good too. Olive oil is also a good fat as it is high in a plant based (but easy to extract) omega 3.

Dairy fats are the next best. Cream, butter and cheese. Next come poultry and animal fats.

Probably less good for you are vegetable oils, sunflower oil, margarines (yes, even the ones which make misleading healthy claims) and worst of all is corn oil (which is used in a lot of fried food and as a standard in the catering industry).

Don't allow the oils and fats to burn. If you overheat any oil it produces *free radicals* which are really bad for you. Don't believe any claims by nutritionists that so-called *anti-oxidant* foods negate free radicals, they simply haven't understood their high-school biology. It's a nice idea - but entirely made up. Don't waste your money. All fried food is bad and any overheated oils are going to do you no favours. If in doubt, stick to an olive oil dressing with your salad and skip everything else.

Dr Phil Harley

Carry water

Carry water. Sip it. It will distract you from hunger.

We don't need to carry water around with us to stay hydrated. This is a myth made up by health-food fanatics who seem to be no healthier than anyone else. You do not need to flush out your kidneys and you do not need the eight magic glasses a day. These are made up myths by nutritionists who have no medical qualifications.

If you dehydrate you will become thirsty. When you are thirsty, go and have a drink. That's it.

There is excellent medical science which says you will not suffer any mental or physical performance loss if you follow this rule.

This applies if you are large, medium or small, if you are young or old, if you are sick or you are well, if you are at school, the office, on the couch or running marathons up sandy hills in the Sahara.

Ok, I've said you don't need to carry water bottles to stay hydrated, but am *still* recommending it. Why?

Good question. Bizarrely, it has now become socially acceptable to carry water. People will barely give you a second glance if you carry a bottle of water with you. Even an enormous one. Buy a big (1.5l) bottle of mineral water. Carry this with you at all times and drink from it often (like a health-food fanatic). When it is empty, refill it from the faucet or tap (there are genuinely no health benefits in mineral water, I promise. There is a reason that *Evian* spelt backwards is naive - I only wish I'd had the idea of putting water into bottles and selling it for a lot of money. I would be on my own Caribbean island already!).

There are some benefits to the carrying of the water. Sipping frequently from this bottle will distract you a little from eating as it gives you something to do. You will be a shade fuller, which will be helpful. You will need to get up to urinate more often (burning an additional few calories). The bottle weighs 1.5kg and this is a mini weights workout to burn another few calories.

It may become your talisman and distract you a little from eating stuff with more calories. It will remind you of your quest. Other people will see and realise you are on your health quest. They will hopefully support your plans.

Please don't buy any electrolyte or other supposed health-giving powders to put in your bottle. Save your money (or send it to me). If you really must put magic powders in, then choose protein powders (the cheapest are as good as the ones with magic sciencey sounding ingredients - choose whey). Unless you have failing kidneys, in which case don't. Apart from providing dietary protein, the other main benefit of protein powders is they can at least help you feel more full. Be aware they taste foul, cost a lot and have calories you might not measure well. But they are a little better for you than eating doughnuts.

Exercise hard

Exercising hard is really good for you.

It helps your muscles stay healthy. It is good for your heart. It gives you better sleep and improved blood flow to the brain. It keeps you fit. It burns lots of calories and decreases hunger.

The body burns extra calories even after the exercise has stopped. These extras are used in repair work, muscle maintenance and replenishing your energy tanks. Getting two sessions of hard exercise a day is ideal but unrealistic in most of our busy lives. If you can manage it, your body, mind and spirit will be grateful.

Exercising hard distracts you from eating both during and after. Hard exercise burns more calories than any other activity, so squeeze it into each and every day that you are able.

Hard exercise releases endorphins. These natural brain chemicals keep you feeling good and healthy for hours after you have finished. You feel happy, alert and your hunger levels are kept right down.

How hard is hard? Enough to hurt a little, enough to make you sweat, enough to make you short of breath. Your self perceived rate of exertion counts. One to ten. Make sure you are at a seven or eight. You should be able to talk within about two minutes of stopping. You should also be able to do an easy session the following day and be ready for another hard one the day after that. If you can't - then you've overdone it. Rest for three days and try again. Keep writing all of this in your diary (at the end of this book - or buy the separate one if you have the digital version).

- *Zero hard sessions a week = declining body state.*
- *One hard session a week = maintenance of current state.*
- *Two hard sessions a week = slow improvement of fitness.*
- *Three hard sessions a week = rapid improvements.*

Being fitter is good because you can then do more during the next exercise session. This is a bonus which makes each session progressively easier to achieve. Over time you are able to do more. Then, when you are able to do more, you get to burn *even* more calories and get to feel *even* better.

Spend a day hungry

Spending a day without any food is something we should all try.

Hungry is only a feeling. Many of us fear it and don't need to.

We should all occasionally try 18 to 24 hours without food. Sometimes. Not very often, just to remind us what it feels like to be hungry. And that it is actually ok. Not pleasant, but nothing to be afraid of.

When you don't eat, you feel hungry. That's it. We have all had this sensation. Sometimes we feel a bit faint. This faint feeling isn't dangerous. This faint feeling is your body trying to get you to go and lie down to conserve your energy stores in case there isn't any more food coming for weeks.

You and I both know that our energy stores contain enough to last for many weeks without anything going in the top end at all.

Many of my patients assume the hunger increases and increases and increase until… They worry about some terrible disaster that may befall them. This is fear of the unknown. Will your head explode, will you go into a coma, will you actually die? They panic.

I don't know what they think might happen. All that does, is that the hunger increases to a maximum point at about fifteen hours after your last meal. It doesn't really change much after that. It goes up and down and you will have some hungry points in your day. If you ignore those and don't eat, the hunger fades again after about half an hour and you forget about being hungry for another hour before it returns. But it goes away again, just the same.

This probably has to be experienced. Because you probably don't believe me. If you are on diabetic medications then don't do this. But there are probably no other excuses not to try it out.

The brain functions perfectly well throughout all of this. Many of my patients assume you can't function well without food. Because the hunger doesn't really go above a certain point, you can even go to sleep on an empty stomach and get a good night's sleep. When you wake, you will be barely more hungry than you would be on any other day. I used to find it remarkable that the brain can deal with hunger like this.

I shouldn't be surprised because the biology makes sense. Hunger is a signal reminding you to go and get food. It makes sense that it fades once it has told you. If you ignore it, the body and brain think you are simply running or walking to go and find some food. So the signal goes quiet. Then it reminds you again in case you have forgotten, before going quiet once more. If there is no food around to be eaten, there would be no point in your body stopping you sleeping or getting enough rest, so it lets you sleep and rest normally. The signal simply reminds you the next morning.

If you were actually running out of food and your brain stopped working well, then you may never find food and could die. So it also makes sense for your brain to work uninterrupted when there is hunger.

It also makes great sense for your body to function at full capacity even when hungry. What would be the point of becoming hungry and then shutting down your muscles, as the body would be unable to seek and find the required food. So what you find is that you can run, jump, climb trees and do all of the stuff you would normally want to be able to do in order to find food. Being hungry doesn't really get in the way of sports performance.

This is all excellent news because if you are wanting a better waistline, you will be wanting to use your body and brain normally. Even when putting fewer calories in the top end, so you can deliberately burn though your excess energy stores. It is really good news that the only thing that will happen is you might feel a bit hungry. So what? Great news indeed.

Growling tummies

When you are hungry, your tummy will growl.

This has a lovely medical word. *Borborygmi*. One borborygmus, two borborygmi. It is the sound of digesting food moving along the gut. Powered by peristaltic waves and gases. Passing from one section to the next as the loops of bowel slide over one another like slippery spaghetti.

It also gives a sensation which is called a hunger pang. It isn't really a pain, it feels different.

Hunger pangs feel different to pain. They are more easily ignored.

Listening to these noises will tell you when you are *actually* hungry. It is nice to know that once they've arrived, they don't really get stronger.

Once your tummy growls, this tells you it would like some food. Just like a pestering pet or an animal it will go quiet after a while if you don't feed it. It takes ten to twenty minutes to fade. After an hour or so, it will remind you again. And so on. It is like your phone alarm or an alarm clock on snooze.

If you would like to eat fewer calories in the day, you should start to ignore these growls. Some of my patients say that they use them to help time their food. Some people like to count to ten of them before they will allow themselves a small healthy snack.

Some people like to listen to the noise, saying it's the sound of hundreds of tiny fat cells bursting. They latch onto this feeling and allow this to encourage them to stay strong and say **no** to the chocolate.

CHAPTER NINE

Muscles move us

Moving more effectively

You are going to die. So am I. So is everyone you and I have ever met. It's just a question of when. I don't know about you, but I am on a personal mission to **fill every remaining minute of my life with nicer and nicer things to do**.

I am also on a mission to **extend my life as much as I possibly can** while I am in good health, so I get more of those precious minutes to enjoy.

I recommend trying these on for size until you find *your own* aims and goals.

How do you want to live the rest of your life? I'm sorry to be blunt but I think it's important. I would love for each day you live to be better than the last. One of the ways to do that is to have a body and brain which are in as good shape as we can get them. Then life feels an awful lot better.

When we move well without pain, when we are strong and supple, when we sleep well and enjoy good sex, life feels good. When we have the company of people we enjoy and get out into the countryside and exercise this brings smiles. I recommend this. I once met a man who told me his life's mission was to find out just how much pleasure the human body could stand. I often think of that and it makes me smile.

Becoming more muscular

Your muscles are fantastic. They really are. Regardless of what size and shape you are now, your muscles as are trainable as anyone else on the planet. This includes very large people, very skinny models and all celebrities. This means international athletes and that person you know who you'd like to be a better shape than.

Having adaptable muscles is a good thing. Modern medical knowledge in the 21st century has some excellent advice for supporting your efforts; *Stretch them, tone them and train them.* They will become stronger, more powerful and more efficient.

Your muscles can be made longer. This means with some careful practice you will be able to touch your toes or whatever it is that you'd like to do . The background science is that the muscles fibers don't actually get longer, but the number of bits that are always contracted and shortened become fewer, the tendon reflexes alter and the range of movement of the nearby joints is increased.

The overall result is greater flexibility. When we become more active it would be nice to get more bang for your buck. Being flexible helps you move and run more efficiently, burn more calories and decreases your chance of getting injured. Injury prevention is really important.

You can get longer muscles, you can get bulkier muscles or you can simply tone what is already there.

Most people find toned muscles desirable. These take a good few weeks of sculpting work. It doesn't all happen overnight. This is a good thing because you can stop before you become too bulky and you can stop before the size of your muscles causes you to do things or lift weights that might cause an injury to an otherwise not very fit system.

Toning your muscles simply involves using them regularly. They will also become more visible when the fat layers currently hiding them become a little bit thinner.

All of these things happen at the same time. The overall effect becomes more visually pleasing as the weeks and months pass by.

Having even slightly bigger muscles is a good thing. Trained muscles have a bigger blood supply, generate more heat and work more efficiently than untrained ones. You can then do more physical work for less apparent effort. It will soon feel easier to run five miles burning 400 calories than it might currently feel to walk two miles briskly.

Having trained muscles burns more calories than having untrained ones. So simply by sitting on the couch or at your desk you will be actively contributing to your beach-ready body mission. Better trained muscles protect your joints better too, with arthritis developing later or minimally. Existing joint pains also heal more quickly.

Having better trained muscles decreases the risk of falling in later life. If you do fall you are less likely to break bones. Staying active is vital as the years progress. This continues to provide benefits into your nineties and beyond. The myth that running and exercise somehow causes your joints to wear out early simply isn't supported by the medical evidence.

There are many and multiple advantages of having better working muscles and these benefits can be gained by pretty much all of us at any point in life, no matter how far things have slid since your early twenties (when most of us were closer to our best).

Moving to be fit

Becoming fit involves more that just getting up and moving about.

What is needed is regular sweaty exercise. Work your body hard enough to build up a sweat and make you short of breath. If you manage this several times a week, you will become fitter and it will become easier. You will live longer by doing this.

To maintain a steady level of health you are recommended to do this for thirty minutes, three times a week. To improve your state of health do even more than this bare minimum.

If you aren't doing this level of sweaty breathless activity (and yes, sex does count - but needs to be for the full thirty minutes) several times a week you are not alone. Many of my patients don't come anywhere close to achieving this level.

* * *

A lot of them feel daunted and give up early. On day one. Before they've even started. I do understand, but they are being silly.

When you start from a low level of fitness, even climbing a flight of stairs can seem like hard work. But the great thing is that the body adapts. You adapt quickly. Your body learns to do what you ask of it. The body will change its very fibers and cells. It will become more able to do breathless, sweaty exercise than you might imagine. It learns to do this at any age. Even my patients in their nineties can learn to move more.

Little by little, bit by bit, day by day. It may take a few weeks or even longer, but it will be do-able. The key is to do a little more each and every day. Your body will respond. And the best news of all is that this will start to feel good.

Sneaky exercise

Every time you do something you burn calories.

The more stuff you do, the more calories you will burn. Sneaky exercise comprises those little things you do that you don't tend to count, all add up and are easy to fit into your day.

There is a nice scientific study on the elderly which shows that *those who fidget, live longer.* Those who can't or won't sit still, live many years longer than those who tend to sit motionless. Moving around is very good for us.

We were designed to use our bodies. If we do not use them, the body and brain start to deteriorate. The great news is that everything counts. Darts, snooker, even reading the paper counts as exercise. Ok, reading the newspaper only counts if you have to walk to the shop to fetch it. But the more you do, the better. Anything.

* * *

If you have the remote control within arm's reach then you aren't going to spend many calories changing the channel. If you keep the remote control on the other side of the room, you will burn a couple. You will work your core muscles getting out of and then back into your chair. Do this. Then think of what else you can sneak into your day. Make it a challenge. Write these small victories down in the diary and try to make them a habit.

Sneaky exercise provides you with a free calorie burn. Sneak tiny bits of exercise into your day whenever you can. Be really smug with yourself every time you manage it. Allow yourself extra smug points any time you could take the easy route but don't. Every time you park a few places further away than you need. Each time you take the stairs rather than the elevator. Every time you walk when you could have used the car. If you take the long route around the supermarket, feel pleased. If you forget something and have to go back for it, this burns calories and should make you smile. Do this, do it every day. Give yourself smug points. Award them every time you do some sneaky exercise.

CHAPTER TEN

Mind games

Managing the mind

Maintaining motivation can be tricky. There are techniques for keeping your motivation levels higher. These are learnable skills. Just like all new skills, you get better at these with more practice.

Lots of people run into psychological speed bumps. These difficulties affect us all to one degree or another.

Overcoming these challenges can be helped by techniques that can be taught or self-taught. Just like techniques to help with motivation, these can be learned. Like other skills, they become easier and more effective the more you practice them.

Every new skill can seem hard or strange at first. But if you work at these, they soon become second nature and eventually require no effort at all. Strangeness gives way to familiarity.

Dr Phil Harley

Managing change

Inertia is one of the fundamental laws of the universe. It is the first law of motion at stated by Sir Isaac Newton: "*An object in motion or at rest will stay in motion or at rest unless another force acts on it.*"

If you didn't take physics or weren't paying that much attention when you did, don't panic. It means: if you are moving you tend to keep going and if you are not then you tend to stay still.

Getting started takes a bit of effort, but once you get going it all becomes relatively easy.

Once you regularly use the stuff here in Skinny Genes it becomes much easier. You can carry on without much effort.

There are two different approaches to getting going. One is the *kick-up-the-bum* method and the other is the *softly-softly* one. They both work and will work on the same person at different times.

The kick-up-the-bum method of getting starting is about making it such a big part of your life that you have to restructure everything else around it. It is simply too big, too massive to ignore.

For example you could decide to run a marathon in the next year. Even if you've never even run for the bus and are about fifty pounds over your ideal bodyweight. Faced with this seemingly impossible task you would have to take a few actions. You might empty your cupboards of unhealthy food, stop all of your daytime snacks, go for a jog at lunchtimes and again after work. You might stop smoking immediately and switch to being teetotal.

This is the *massive motivation, huge goals, big kick-up-the-bum method* and is **very** effective. This is about making the goal seem so very large, almost impossible and you then commit to actually doing it. You will then have no choice other than to make the most of your waking moments. This will hopefully put you right off eating junk food and snacks. You may then start to make sensible food and exercise choices to support you in your quest.

If that strategy scares you (and it should, that is the whole point of how it works) then maybe the *softly-softly* approach could be more up your street (at the moment anyway). The softly-softly approach to change is all about making the changes so small that they seem achievable.

For example you could make yourself walk twenty extra steps

today and could leave one bite of your lunch on the plate. You might also drink one glass of water before your evening meal.

These changes are probably within the grasp of even the most committed couch potato. The idea here is that the next day you do the same as the previous day and add in something else. Something small and achievable. Maybe eating one fewer candy bar (or only eating half) and substituting a piece of whole fruit.

One of the keys to getting this method to work is to write stuff down when you do it. This yields a happiness boost of endorphins, giving you a mental gold star. This reward system is of course inside your head but it works. It works even though the reward is pretend and all you've done is write it down. It can be in your journal, on your smart-phone or on the back of an envelope. It is the action and then the writing it down which is key.

To enhance the kick-up-the-bum method, make a public commitment. Tell everyone your goal. Friends, family, neighbors, work colleagues. Ask them to badger you about it day in and day out until it is done. People are usually more than pleased to be able to help. Some of them may enjoy nagging you.

If you succeed you will inspire them and they will shower you with congratulations. If you fail they will feel smug. Don't let that bother you as they haven't been bothered to do anything quite so ballsy. Either way, they will be fascinated with how you are progressing and this can be highly motivating.

Dr Phil Harley

Smart goals and motivation

SMART goals work because they are smart. A lot is talked about goals. A goal is an arbitrary thing you decide that you want. You get to pick. Some people's goals could be:

- I'd like to be a size ten.

- I'd like to be skinny.

- I'd like to look great naked.

- I'd like to be buff.

- I'd like to run a half marathon.

- I'd like my knees to hurt less.

With goals we can use psychology to help them be more achievable. Our brains are specifically geared towards getting us to do stuff. Humans are naturally goal driven and in Skinny Genes we will use the best brain tools for the job.

* * *

SMART goals are: Specific, Measurable, Achievable, Realistic and Time defined.

SMART goals have the bonus of tending to get done. If your goals aren't SMART they don't tend to actually happen. It is for this reason we are going to take the time to carefully aim our brain before we fire.

Try writing your goals down. Take a large piece of paper, write them in the middle and scribble ideas around the outside. An example could be:

- I would like to run a half marathon - **specific**.
- **Measurable** - I will know I've achieved this because I will have a medal and a photo of me looking sweaty.
- This is **achievable** as I can already walk six miles in an afternoon.
- **Realistic** - lots of other people can do that and I'm not very different to them.
- **Time defined** - I will do this at the local half marathon in six months time.

A less good example of a SMART goal could be:

- I'd like to be slim.
- This is less likely to happen and that would be a shame. Not SMART.
- It is not **specific** (how slim? what is slim?).
- What are you **measuring**? (waist size, able to do up your jeans, number of chins? - if you know, then say so).

- **Achievable** - most things are achievable, but at a maximum speed that you will get a feel for. Ten dress sizes in a week probably isn't achievable in that time frame.

- **Realistic** - I'm never going to be professional gymnast or a ballet dancer, but I might be able to run faster than everyone in my street.

- **Time defined** - if your goal is open ended with no defined end point then you will find it much easier to put off doing anything about it. There will be no sense of urgency and you are less likely to feel you are on a mission to achieve your goal. Having this sense of purpose is critical.

- A time target is important (you are allowed to shift the goalposts later, but at the beginning you should be specific). If you do not mark out your time frame, you will tend to procrastinate and put off your actions for another day.

Why not write down a SMART goal. I'll wait for you.

Done?

Maintaining momentum

There will inevitably be times when we need to adjust our goals. Life has a tendency to simply get in the way and that is ok. We will cope with the occasional extra obstacle, hurdle or stepping stone on our journey to success.

We can revise our goals up, down or we can re-write them entirely. Reset and start again. If our goals are too small there is the danger they will not motivate us to action (*lose one pound over the next fifteen years*) and if too large and apparently unobtainable they won't inspire us to action (*be the lead backing dancer for Beyoncé on her next world tour*). If you find that you are stuck and not moving forward, then revisiting your goals and tinkering a little can be very helpful.

Maintaining motivation can be a challenge for all of us. Motivation can wane. I know this piece of news may be shocking, but I have on occasion felt that I really can't be arsed and I'd rather sit on the couch eating cookies and inhaling popcorn. Let's face it, we are all human and sometimes motivation for the future doesn't really come close to the power of the instant gratification of the here and now. This is quite normal and there is good psychological research to back this up (on hyperbolic discounting).

Parts of our brain are hardwired to do this unhelpful thinking. This doesn't make it a good excuse. It's just to say that there is no blame attached to taking a wrong turn every now and again.

The key is noticing when we are off track and in then turning back to point in the right direction. Motivating ourselves to keep making smart choices, taking a step or two each day in the correct direction takes some doing. Staying focused and on track is the key. You already know most of what needs to be done. Just because it is simple, that doesn't make it easy.

Keep your eyes on the prize and keep your feet moving.

Make each day about what **you** want. If it is someone else's goal you are less likely to do as well. You are much more likely to rebel. At least if you are anything like me you will. To rebel against an authority telling you what to do is a natural instinct, a survival based emotion and a perfectly natural response.

So make the goals about **you**, have something that **you** really want. Make it achievable and check in with it each day. If it looms too large, break it down into manageable bite sized chunks. Write them down in an ordered list. Have the next item on the list as your next goal. Then the next and so on.

Motivation fades a bit for all of us. It wanes even faster in the face of temptation. Temptation wouldn't be the same if it wasn't tempting. Help yourself on your journey by keeping your plans flexible. Adjust them as you go along. Have lots of different actions which will help you towards your goals. You get to pick a different one each day for variety, or if life events take over and stop you doing one of them. Keeping checking in to see how you are doing. Get feedback on your progress. Loop this back into your next actions. These steps will move you forward. Each and every day.

Rather than trying to manage all of the steps 100% better (as this might prove a bigger challenge than we are ready for), try and do one hundred things 1% better. After a few weeks try and improve another 1%. Before you know it you will find yourself making real progress. More on this in the tips section.

Setting yourself rules to follow is part of most success stories with the Skinny Genes plan. Rules that only you will know if you break them.

The great thing with making up rules is that *you* are only accountable to *you*. Only you and no one else. You get to decide. You set the rule, you set its limits, you decide on exceptions to the rules. You get to suspend the rules for special occasions. You get to choose about having a piggy bank that you load with a dollar, pound or euro each time you break them (if that sort of thing motivates you).

* * *

Some of my patients get on well with *star-charts*. Ten days with a star = reward / treat. You get to decide what earns a star, how many stars you need and what the treat will be. This works best if you actually stick small gold stars on a big piece of paper on your refrigerator.

Goal setting

When you decide stuff you become motivated. You feel like you can achieve anything.

If you are anything like me, that lasts for about five minutes. The good intentions fade fast. The shiny vision of what you just know to be your best path fades against the brighter image of the sofa, the power of the duvet, the horror of the rainy day and the fatal lure of the snack cupboard.

You vow to try again tomorrow.

Realize you are fallible, human and normal. Work with this.

Build in contingency plans. What will you do when you bump up against some obstacles? The best thing is probably to simply accept them for what they are. Irritations you would rather not have. Roll with the punches. Pick yourself up, dust yourself off and carry on. Each day you wake, you get a brand shiny new day to play with. Hope starts afresh each morning. Zig Ziglar is quoted:

"People often say that motivation doesn't last. Well, neither does bathing, that's why we recommend it daily."

Plan ahead with your head. Realistically you will need some down-time. Accept this. Recharging and zoning out are normal. Plan to fail a bit each day. If you do, you will be ok with that and if you don't, you get to feel really pleased with yourself. Well done you, you clever sausage.

Aim high but be realistic in what you anticipate you can manage each day. The key here is simply to think about what you are doing and how you are making bits of progress each day. Having your motivating goal to hand is a great help in making good decisions, moment by moment and day by day.

CHAPTER ELEVEN

Need nudging?

Snacking control

Snacking control is about controlling availability and hunger urges.

A major part of snacking control is about availability:

- *Availability of motivation around consequences.*
- *Availability of other options.*
- *Availability of snacks.*
- *Availability of time to snack.*

Motivation around consequences - this is about thinking through what the snack will bring for you. Sure, the chocolate will taste nice, I'm not denying that. But you've entered a marathon and every bit of choccy will make it just that bit harder in the final few miles. Is it really worth it? Is it worth the tiny tastebud pleasure?

* * *

You alone can answer this. Develop the important habit of asking yourself the question and answering honestly. *Do I really want this?*

Are there other options than the unhealthy thing in front of me? This also depends on why you are snacking. If you are **bored** you should think of something else to go and do. If you are hungry then try some water or choose a low calorie filling-up kind of snack. If you are **sad** then snacking is really not a good strategy as you could probably consume your own bodyweight without too much effort. Am I about to eat this because it is convenient and in front of me? Would I be better off making a scrumptious salad, full of fresh healthy tasty food to nourish my body and soul?

Having the snacks less available is a big one. I recommend emptying your cupboards of snacks. Empty your bag, purge your purse, clear your work drawers and your car. Remove temptation wherever possible.

STOP buying snacks.

Buy no booze, buy no sweets, buy no crisps, chips or dips. Forget about muffins, cookies, pastries and doughnuts. Become a stranger to chocolate entirely.

If the snacks are not there and obtaining them involves a journey to fetch them, this adds a helpful layer of complexity to the process. You might see sense before the deed is done and actually not go through with your frenzied plan to obtain and eat all the snacks you can carry from the convenience store.

* * *

Do NOT go shopping when you are hungry.

Having the available time to snack is crucial to putting the calories in. If you are on a sinking ship and bailing frantically to keep afloat you are not likely to work your way through any snacks, even if they were within arm's reach. If you are watching a movie at the cinema …Ok, bad example. If you are reading the world's best book, or are in bed with the person or persons of your dreams (real or imagined) you are less likely to reach for a snack. Driving a car at high speed down narrow streets, chased by gangsters is not going to be a journey full of snacking.

Car journeys are full of opportunities to gorge on calorie dense foods. The chocolate industry turns over billions every year and the majority of this is bought at gas stations. This is why there is so much variety available every time you fill up with fuel. Having it there works. And don't get me started on drive-throughs.

I rail against these for a couple of reasons. The first reason is that we will struggle to get great waist management without any additional temptations. The second is that billions a year is a lot of money and frankly I'm jealous. It's high time that you and I reclaimed some of this money as our own. Start today!

Part of snacking control is around hunger signals and pre-empting them. Nip it in the bud. Get the snack in early if you are going to have the snack anyway. Have a smaller snack early rather than a less well controlled snacking episode later. Eating little and often so as not to become hungry is a technique often talked about and has some merit.

Don't forget delayed gratification.

Delayed gratification is the fancy term used when we wait for the pleasure. When we are made to wait or get someone else to wait just that bit longer for the pleasure (this can be food along with various other things that I'm sure you could think of if you concentrate and really put your mind to it) - when the pleasure or gratification is delayed it seems just that extra bit special. The waiting can be a good feeling and the delicious anticipation might sometimes be almost as good as the resolution of the experience.

If you force yourself to wait, you will enjoy it all the more when it comes. This applies to snacks too. In one of Terry Pratchett's excellent books in the Discworld fantasy series, one of the witches has written a book called 'The Joy of Snacks'. Using a delayed gratification strategy brings its own rewards.

Don't underestimate the brain boost given by nature. Go for a walk in the woods, by the beach, canal, along a river, around a park or any other green space where nature is. The benefit to your wellbeing is in addition to the delaying and offsetting hunger bonus the exercise gives. Going for a walk or a run outside will be *sooo* much better for you than eating the family pack of potato chips currently eagerly clutched in your paw.

I had a patient tell me how well she'd been doing. She'd tried for ages to eat smaller portions and eat them more slowly. When she fell off the wagon she turned to me with a sad face and said '*I'm afraid I just went piraña*'. She described how she would Hoover the food like a demented twister. Anything nearby was consumed in a sort of feeding frenzy.

I sympathize. I too have inhaled food without thinking. Immediately followed by remorse. Struck by that sinking feeling of having undone all the good I'd previously achieved.

It's important to realize it happens to all us from time to time. The trick is to make is happen progressively less often. Ideally not every day anyway!

Procrastinating

Snacking out of boredom happens. As humans we are also prone to absent minded snacking.

You and I probably both reach for snacks when we are a little bit bored. If you are bored I want you to start to recognize this for what it is. It's not bad to be bored and you are welcome to it if that's what you like. However, it is a big risk factor for snacking.

Going to the shops, rummaging through the cupboards and checking the fridge when you are bored will often end in non-necessary snacking and non-helpful excess calories. If you find yourself in this position and notice, give yourself a pat on the back for noticing. Awareness of this doesn't come easily at first, though the benefits are great. When you notice you are bored, immediate action and busy-ness is required. Go and do something (anything) and you will soon discover the snacking urge can be postponed, quietened down (or even forgotten entirely).

If you are watching a film or your favourite soap, or chatting to friends over a drink in a bar there is a tendency to graze. The hands put food in your face, often without engaging the brain.

The danger with this is these foods are often high calorie or deep fried. Because this grazing is not driven by hunger the fullness stop signal doesn't arrive. Because the brain is distracted it doesn't easily tell you to slow the intake down. A common unhelpful habit is to always eat popcorn and ice cream when watching a movie.

In the Skinny Genes plan it isn't that you can't have popcorn or ice cream, it's just that we should learn to be aware of what we are doing and don't accidentally undo a whole lot of our good work.

Mastering control over our snacking plays a big part in gaining control over our destiny. Snacking from time to time can be very nice. But the key is that we do this out of choice and with awareness.

Snacking to delay getting on with stuff = nibbly procrastination.

Nibbly procrastination is delaying getting on with a task by grazing on food, cruising the cupboards and generally scoffing what you might end up regretting thirty minutes later. This is unhelpful. Nothing gets achieved and unnecessary calories go in.

Most of us procrastinate more than we perhaps would like to. Sorting this out is a whole other book (**Do it, Do it. Do it!** - A

Procrastinator's Guide to World Domination. Out soon. Though ones by other authors are probably also available).

Packed lunch

If you plan and prepare your lunchtime meals in advance you can better control your calorie intake. You can think about putting less spread on the bread, choosing high fiber options, adding less mayonnaise and so on. You can even make a large batch in advance.

Batch making gives lots of identical meals which can then be frozen. Having identical meals gives food boredom and one is less likely to eat enthusiastically - which in terms of the Skinny Genes plan is a good thing. A little dull perhaps, but probably worth it in your quest for a beach-ready body.

Removing frozen sandwiches on the day of eating means they won't be edible before lunchtime and decreases the chance that you will consume them before the hour for luncheon arrives.

Tips to delay your morning snacks include going for a short

walk, chewing sugar-free gum and sipping slowly a glass of water, tea or coffee. Don't forget, the milk in tea and coffee contains calories too. Try taking it black or have skimmed fat-free milk.

The way you make your tea and coffee is part of effective waist management.

Tea and coffee should be taken without sugar. If you choose to add milk then make this skimmed and fat-free. Additionally they should be taken early enough in the day so the caffeine doesn't prevent you getting a really good night's sleep. Getting good quality rest is crucial.

I suggest not using artificial sweeteners as this contributes to your sweet tooth habit. The habit of enjoying and rewarding yourself with sweet tasting stuff is not going to do you any long term favors. When you are tired and faced with a choice between sweet or savory, you are more likely to choose sweet if that is your habit. This will usually contain more calories. The calories all add up over a lifetime.

Whichever way you currently take your tea or coffee, you can adjust to having no sugar and skimmed fat-free milk within about three weeks. This is how long your tastebuds and the brain wiring from these signals takes to fully adjust. Make the change today and wait - it will work. You will come to enjoy your new version just as much. It will be so much better for you and will not hamper your other efforts in your brilliant Skinny Genes plan.

Go easy on the sauce

Less alcohol is better for a number of reasons. Less snacking, more food enjoyment, fewer calories, less adverse effect on the next day's exercise and less blunted awareness of quite how much food you are actually eating.

If you don't have alcohol with your meal then you won't want to snack as much later. Alcohol does genuinely drop your blood sugar a bit. This is one of the reasons why it makes you munch. When you do eat, your mental resistance is lowered and you may eat more and choose less well than if you didn't have any alcohol on board.

If you have alcohol in your system your senses will be blunted. Your enjoyment of the food is impaired as your taste is less sensitive. These are wasted calories. *I'm not enjoying it, but the calories are still accumulating.* You are less able to judge the full signal and may eat more than you need or actually really want.

* * *

Booze in your body takes a while to process. Your body treats it as a poison and eliminates this toxin. It is broken down at a steady rate by the liver and the byproducts are lost in urine, feces, sweat and on the breath. Going through this process feels unpleasant and makes you less enthusiastic about most things (the hangover effect). Exercise is one of those things. A drink today will make you significantly less likely to exercise efficiently tomorrow.

This is ok from time to time. If you think about it and are aware of what you are doing then I'm very happy for you to do whatever pleases you. You are a grown up. Just be careful about doing it without thinking through the implications.

The power of sleep

When we get a good night's sleep, everything else becomes easier. Your slimmer trimmer waist quest is aided and supported by sleeping well.

Some scientific progress is being made in understanding sleep in terms of the hunger hormones *ghrelin* and *leptin*. These are affected by sleep deprivation. In murine studies they affect weight gain and satiety (how much the mouse eats before it is full). There is more progress to be made. What we do know for certain is:

Sleep is good. Sleep is important. Sleep keeps us healthy.

- If we do not get enough sleep we overeat.
- If we do not get enough rest, our willpower is lower.
- If we do not get enough sleep we put on weight.

- If we put on weight this will result in poorer quality sleep.

Whatever you need to do to get a good night's sleep then do it. Caffeine will not help. This can stay in your system for many hours. Most people need zero caffeine after midday to function at their best.

Having a bedtime routine is helpful. Avoid over-stimulation before sleep. I mean electronic devices, television, internet and email. Over-bright rooms with artificial light can impair the quality of our sleep. We sleep better with a period of winding down. This is helped by mood lighting or a good book. Pyjamas, a snuggle, a mug of (low-cal) cocoa and then off to brush your teeth.

Five portions a day

The authorities (lead by the reputable *World Health Organisation*) say that we should eat five portions a day of vegetables or fruit. The original research found the actual number was higher (closer to ten), but it was felt the public wasn't ready to hear the truth. That was ten years ago.

If we eat too much fruit we will take too many calories onboard (not to mention heartburn and loose bowels). Eat two pieces of whole-fruit a day and make the rest up with vegetables. There is probably no upper limit on the benefit to your Skinny Genes plan of eating more vegetables.

Frozen vegetables are cheap, widely available and conveniently stay fresh. Sometimes cheaper than fresh produce, they can be cooked from frozen in only a few minutes. Stuff your freezers with all the varieties you can find (and eat them daily).

* * *

If you can manage seven veggie portions a day, this will be excellent for your waist plan. Cook them any way you like, apart from roasting or frying in high calorie oils. If you boil them, you should note that all the healthy vitamin C (ascorbic acid) leaks out into the water. If you don't want that, either drink the water or choose an alternative cooking method.

One hundred percent

Wanting to do something one hundred percent better may be daunting and can seem impossible.

Accurate mathematics aside, if you do one hundred things one percent better, this is just as good and easier to achieve. One hundred percent improvement, minimal effort. Try it. Maybe try one a day …

One hundred things to try one percent better this week.

1. Walk faster.
2. Go for a jog.
3. Park further away.
4. Sit up straight.
5. Stand well without slouching.
6. Take a glass of water with your meals.

7. Eat whole-wheat choices.

8. Two pieces of whole-fruit a day.

9. Don't finish your plate.

10. Put your cutlery down between each mouthful.

11. Chew more, eat slowly (enjoy it).

12. Drink less alcohol.

13. Get enough sleep.

14. Don't go shopping when you are hungry.

15. Don't buy snacks at the checkout.

16. Don't buy snacks at the gas station.

17. Journal your food intake.

18. Write your goals down.

19. Choose smaller plates.

20. Don't have a second portion.

21. Have a larger portion of vegetables.

22. Something green with every meal.

23. Choose leaner meats.

24. Trim the fat from your meat.

25. Choose a lower fat spread.

26. Select skimmed fat-free milk.

27. Take no sugar in tea or coffee.

28. Choose sugar-free squash or cordial.

29. Add less oil to your cooking.

30. Make your own meals. No ready meals, no more TV dinners.

31. Don't have any fast-food, nothing from a drive-through.

32. Eat fewer nachos or potato chips as snacks.

33. Don't skip breakfast.

34.   Ignore the hunger pangs until you can hear them.

35.   Don't snack when you are bored.

36.   Don't snack when you aren't concentrating on the food (TV, Internet *et cetera*).

37.   Zero fries.

38.   No sodas. No fizzy or carbonated drinks.

39.   ...

Ok, I do know there aren't a hundred. But I will stick my neck out and say that if you can conquer this lot, then you are well on your way. Let's see if you can make a one percent improvement on how you are doing the above things this week.

The great thing about one percent is you get to decide quite how much that is and you can make this quite do-able.

Come back to the list at the end of the week and have a think how you are getting on. There are no judgments to be made, no beating yourself up. Simply congratulate yourself on any progress and next week have a go at improving all those things another one percent.

Snack control tips

Snack control tips. Follow them.

THINk about what you are eating.

- Lots and lots of vegetables.
- Water with meals.
- No alcohol before the evening meal has finished.
- No snack availability with alcohol.
- Have two courses only.
- Don't finish your plate.
- Don't finish anyone else's plate.
- Don't tidy up the serving bowl or roasting tray.
- Sugar-free squash not high juice.
- Water not fruit juice.

- Skimmed fat-free milk.

- No sugar in tea or coffee.

- No cookies. No pretzels. No chips.

- No sodas or fizzy drinks.

- Fewer fries.

- Don't choose fried anything.

- Two pieces of whole-fruit each day.

- Beware the goggle box (TV).

- Less chocolate.

- Don't eat food that you like.

- Eat expensive food.

- No processed food.

Lots and lots of vegetables

Vegetables are full of goodness, plenty of fiber, are cheap, crammed with flavor, few calories, their bulk will help fill you up and their high protein content will keep you full. I cannot over-stress the benefits of having lots of veg each and every day.

Salad isn't quite as good. Due to its high water content it munches down to nothing and lots of it contains natural sugars which have calories you might not notice. Vegetable crisps are not so good either. They are very high in calories due to the oil they are cooked in and having the same energy content as normal chips (crisps in the UK). You might feel virtuous eating them but you will be poorer and probably no thinner.

* * *

It's all about eating actual vegetables. Preferably not fried or roasted, as oil is very high in calories.

Water with meals

Filling up with water is a cheap trick. It's cheap and it's a trick. But worth weaving in as it does help a little. It is also better for you than drinking alcohol.

No alcohol before the evening meal has finished

This delays the need for alcohol and hopefully you will drink less, or even none at all.

No snack availability with alcohol

If you do drink alcohol, do not eat bar snacks, don't go for a curry, nor a Chinese, tacos, pizza or burger and fries on the way home. You will eat more than you require (because your judgment is impaired) and seriously, when else do you find the need for a meal on the way home at one in the morning? Trust me, you don't really need to eat. You need two glasses of water and put yourself to bed.

Have two courses only

When you are in a restaurant two courses are probably enough. Have a starter and main or main and pudding. Try to get out of the habit of eating so much that it hurts. That doesn't support your Skinny Genes plans at all.

Don't finish your plate

Eat like the Queen of England. She apparently leaves a morsel. A lone forkful remains on her plate. This says to whomever is feeding her; *'That was delicious but I don't require any more, thank you so very much'*. Otherwise her plate would be filled again and etiquette would compel her to finish that one too, and so on.

Leaving food on our plate is hard for a lot of us as many of our parents and their parents were taught to always finish your plate each and every time. *Think of the starving children* and so on. This was understandable but I don't care about understandable. I want Skinny Genes to help you look better naked in front of the mirror. It is time for new habits: **Smaller plates, smaller portions and don't finish everything**. This is the new way. If you don't alter your ways, your waist may not alter.

Leave a little bit, this will also encourage you to put less on your plate next time. There is good science to prove that having smaller plates helps you to eat less. Choose side plates rather than your biggest plate. Your brain then thinks you have a big portion when it fills the smaller plate. I don't personally know how my brain could be fooled by something so simple and I'm bit ashamed that it is - but the good news is that it works regardless. Try it.

Don't finish anyone else's plate

Don't be an oinker, you've usually eaten quite enough. Don't forget to wait twenty minutes for the tummy full signal to arrive.

Don't tidy up the serving bowl or roasting tray

It's ok to throw food away and certainly better than putting on unnecessary weight. If it makes you feel that bad, then make less next time. The same goes for tidying up your children's leftovers. That is not ok if you then eat your own meal. Put it into the trash or buy a goat. Stop eating it.

Sugar-free squash not high juice

This is an easy choice, do you add in calories or not? Choose the one with no calories. The sugar-free versions taste pretty good but if you don't like the taste, choose water.

Water not fruit juice

This is the same as the point above. Fruit juice has no fiber and about 400 calories in a glass. Water has no calories.

Skimmed fat-free milk

You should get out of the habit of drinking anything other than skimmed fat-free milk. You do not need the fat. There is nothing good about it and it turns a high protein drink with lots of calcium into a fatty drink with far too many calories.

It takes only a few weeks to get used to the new taste. Do it. Don't delay. After a month or so it will feel strange if you are given anything else. You will probably live longer for making just this simple small choice.

No sugar in tea or coffee

This is like making the switch to skimmed fat-free milk. Do it. Do it now. Your taste preferences will adjust quickly no matter how long you've taken sugar for and no matter how strange it seems at first. It is very easy to pack a lot of extra calories in quickly by added sugar.

No cookies. No pretzels. No chips

You do not need cookies, pretzels or potato chips in your life. Learn to do without these snacks. There are plenty of other things on the supermarket shelves to eat and these snacks are particularly low in anything resembling nutrition. It is too easy to eat lots and lots of calories here without thinking very much and that is not going to help your Skinny Genes plan.

No sodas or fizzy drinks

Sodas and fizzy drinks can be excluded from the diet. Completely. They contain no nutrition and most of them come in a high calorie version which it is all too easy to buy and drink. If you do not routinely drink them then resisting that bit of temptation is that much easier. Drop the soda.

There is science research showing that people who drink diet-cola are more likely to put on weight than if they drink the full-fat version. This is likely to be the type of people who are doing the choosing rather than the drinks being bad, but if you avoid all carbonated drinks you avoid the problem completely.

Sweetened fizzy drinks are going to keep your sweet tooth going. This isn't going to help you in the long term. Sweet fizzy drinks are manufactured to appeal to children. You are a grownup. Managing your waistline may need grownup strategies.

Fewer fries

Fries taste nice to most of us. Few of us would want to cut them out completely. Having oven chips is a little better as they have less calorie laden oil but they don't taste as nice as their fatty relations. This means that chips or fries are pretty incompatible with a Skinny

Genes plan.

If you must have them, then have fewer. Don't eat them every day. Twice a month would be reasonable. Do not eat a whole portion. Share it. A regular portion.

Don't choose fried anything

When choosing your food, try to get into the habit of choosing an option which isn't fried. When eating out there is often a choice, choose the non-fried. This too will eventually become a habit. Fried food is one of those tastes which after a while of not eating it you seem to miss less and less. This is a good thing.

Two pieces of whole-fruit each day

Fruit contains a lot of sugar. It also contains fiber and fills you up reasonably. This is acceptable as a snack. A glass of smoothie contains the same or more calories but no fiber. This is super-high in sugars and is best avoided. It is reasonable to eat two pieces of fruit a day. This satisfies your desire for sweet things in a way that involves a lot fewer calories than cookies, chocolate or cake.

Beware the goggle box (TV)

Do not eat anything in front of the television, laptop or anything you can access Facebook on.

I appreciate this may come across as a little harsh but I think you get the point. In front of the TV a lot-cal hot chocolate is acceptable, little else is.

Less chocolate

If you must eat chocolate then choose prohibitively expensive versions (such as *Godiva* from Belgium) and really savor just one or two pieces.

Try to get out of the habit of buying or eating chocolate most days. It should be relegated, or elevated depending on your point of view to a once weekly or even fortnightly treat.

Don't eat food that you like

If you enjoy what is in front of you, it is likely to get eaten. This isn't complex but consider a small boy. What is the difference between snot-boogers and cabbage? The answer is that an unattended small boy probably wouldn't eat the cabbage.

If you don't enjoy a food or even actively dislike it you may place less on your plate, are less likely to finish it and will thus achieve a master-stroke towards excellent waistline management.

Eat expensive food

If all you eat is *Beluga* caviar, you might not be able to afford much of this. You will thus be more reluctant to pile this on your plate as you may need a second mortgage before too long.

I appreciate that caviar might not be your thing but I'm sure you get the idea.

No processed food

This is important. By making your own food you gain complete control over what goes in. You will think about and may even modify your meals to best suit your plan. You will probably add less fat and less sugar than comes in pre-packed meals. You will be more likely to eat it at a table rather than on your knee in front of the TV. This slows eating and helps make it conscious. Again, this is a good thing.

Stuck checklist

The Skinny Genes checklist for when you feel a bit stuck

- Why do you want a better waist?

- What is it about managing your waistline that would feel great?

- What do you want to be able to say to yourself when you see your reflection?

- Imagine the next few months going perfectly, what will that look like?

- When you have a good day, how pleased with yourself do you feel?

- If I eat this will I be pleased with myself tonight? (DIET = Did I Eat That)

- Does that piece of food look like good fuel to put into a healthy body?

- Would an Olympic athlete be healthier if they ate that?

- Is this going to be a plus point or a minus point for an amazing body?

- Will I look sexier if I do this?

- Is there some green in this meal?

- Have I eaten two pieces of fruit today?

- Have I left the house today for some exercise?

- Am I getting a good night's sleep?

- Have I cut down on afternoon caffeine and is my alcohol intake low enough?

- Have I cut down all my fizzy drinks?

- Am I getting enough vegetables?

- Have I stopped adding sugar to food and drink?

- Are my portion sizes too big?

- Am I eating slowly enough?

- Do I have a glass of water with every meal?

- Am I eating when I'm actually a little bit thirsty?

- Am I snacking when I'm distracted?

- Am I eating because I'm bored, lonely, unhappy, stressed or procrastinating?

- Is there a sports star, film star or celebrity I look up to, who would endorse this next snack I'm contemplating?

- What would my favourite celebrity do?

- Am I really hungry or is this simply habit?

- Will I actually enjoy this, *really really* enjoy this and feel good afterwards? (If the answer is yes, then go for it, you've got it nailed.)

- Am I keeping a journal of the calories in and the daily activities?

- Am I being realistic and totally honest in my journal?

- Do I write in my journal and workbook everyday?

- Which quotes inspire me?

- On my fridge, is there a hero picture or is it Miss Piggy?

- Is this food ok for a caveman?

- Does this food need a label to identify it?

- Is there anything fried in this meal?

- Are these healthy fats?

- Are any of these fats non-natural?

- Is this going to make me trim, slim and sexy?

- Is this going to make me healthier or less healthy? You will almost certainly know. If on the rare occasion you can't figure it out ...Then don't eat it. It really is that simple. Nice and easy does it, eat stuff that's good for you, don't eat too much. Eat it slowly, enjoy it. Get lots of good sleep and healthy outdoors exercise. Repeat every day and strip off to inspect the progress in a mirror.

CHAPTER TWELVE

Tying it together

Summary

The end of this and the start of your new beginning ...

What are the steps in Skinny Genes?

- Accept your body's biology will make you fat unless you concentrate hard and make a bit of an effort.
- Learn what hunger is and what it isn't.
- Make better food choices each and every day.
- Use your body the best way that you can. Keep yourself fit and active.
- Sleep well. Rest and recuperation are part of a healthy life.
- Recognize snacking for what it is - unnecessary calories and best avoided.
- Keep busy and focused working towards SMART goals.

- Keep a journal of progress, calories in and exercise done, along with daily thoughts.

- Change lifelong habits around food. This is very achievable, worth doing and takes about two months.

- Changes feel strange at first like new shoes, but become automatic and comfortable with time.

The body is well adapted for an environment which we no longer live in. The body and brain sometimes need some help in selecting the best choices. In previous times Mother Nature had a way of helping us make the best choices. Calories were scarce, there were no comfy chairs and our only transport was to walk or run.

Now we live in such comfortable times that we need more help. We have no mental difficulty in controlling what children do for their own good. Adults still need help. We choose cheesecake over a raw turnip and this is quite natural. It's ok to want the cheeseburger over the crab apple but it doesn't make it particularly good for us.

Children don't know enough to be able to make good choices in life, so we help them by setting rules such as not selling them cigarettes. We stop them drinking alcohol. It may be that the poor decision-making skills and poor judgement-calls of children don't improve much as we grow up.

Adults are at risk of making some pretty unhelpful choices. Once we accept this, we can work with it. If someone is making a series of unhelpful choices they can end up making a mess of whatever it is they were trying to do.

* * *

We often make food choices that are not as supportive for our future health as they could be. It is a natural tendency to make decisions about the short term (*this doughnut is going to taste pretty yummy and I'm feeling hungry*) while discounting the long term effects (*when I'm so heavy that my knees hurt I may regret some of the doughnuts*).

The longer the delay between the action and the consequences, the easier it is to discount. Even something the next day is easy to ignore as a human. For example if I have more than one alcoholic drink I don't feel good the next day, if I have more than two I feel unwell. Yet after the first drink, all I want is another one as it feels so good. I find it difficult to stop at one even though I'm fully aware of the consequences and know that I would regret it.

When we make food decisions it is weeks, months and years before the effects are felt, so it is no wonder that making better choices proves tricky.

Educating people about what to eat isn't enough, it is important to point out the elephant in the room. It isn't natural to choose healthy food when you have high fat, high calorie options available.

The bad stuff tastes good.

We all like it. But that's not the point. We need to find ways and strategies for making better choices.

Our tastes and the desire for certain foods change over our

lifetimes. Children don't like Brussels sprouts, and only grownups seem to like olives. One of the reasons our tastebuds seem to change may be due to changes in the bacteria that inhabit our gut.

We live in harmony with ten billion bacteria. There are ten times more bacteria in and on you than the number of human cells you have. Somewhere between one and three percent of your body mass is bacteria. This is known as the human microbiome.

In our digestive tracts thousands of different bacteria species help us digest food. The populations will vary from time to time and this helps explain why we select the foods we do. When we deliberately avoid a food and reintroduce it weeks later, we no longer enjoy it as much and the desire for it fades.

This is partly the psychological shift of habit change. It is also likely that the relative populations of bacteria have shifted. Hopefully in a way that assists you with changing from full-cream to skimmed fat-free milk, from chocolate to carrots, from cake to celery and from fruit juice to whole-fruit.

After a while you will genuinely start to enjoy and want the new choices. The very best bit about this shift is that you can choose to do it deliberately.

Good luck. Keep up the good work and keep making better choices every day.

About the Author

Thank you for reading my book

If you enjoyed this, I would very much appreciate you leaving feedback on the online store website.

Sign up today at www.brainsolutions.co.uk for:

20 daily tips - FREE daily emails to give you a boost in your Waist Management

_____

About the author

Dr Harley lives and works in the South of the UK with his family.

In his spare time he reads more about running than is probably good for him.

He's told he should get out more (though he obviously think that means on the trails).

A General Practitioner in the UK for over ten years, he has a special interest in weight management.

Sign up for his free 20 daily tips email if you'd like to hear more about tips about how to manage your waist.

If you have feedback, comments, questions or suggestions, please email phil@brainsolutions.co.uk

_____

This book works a lot better if you complete a journal. The print version has a diary section at the back lovingly crafted by me. It will really help you to complete this or something like it. It's all about the Hawthorne effect.

You can purchase follow-on diaries online at all good stores, including:

Www.brainsolutions.co.uk

_____

Check out brainsolutions.co.uk for more titles by Dr Phil Harley

coming soon ...

* * *

BetterDay - stress management for busy people

Desert Marathon Training - a beginners guide to one of the world's toughest footraces; *The Marathon des Sables (Out Now)*

Beginners guide to running

Do it, *do it*, DO IT! - A Procastinator's Guide to World Domination

CHAPTER THIRTEEN

Workbook

How to use it

The workbook may be your most helpful section. Use it daily to support your progress. It will work best if you complete all of the sections.

The system here in Skinny Genes is about eating well, moving well and managing hunger. This is best done by creating supportive habits. Automatic behaviors which help you make better decisions.

Better choices. Every day.

It is sixty days long and designed to help you establish the best new habits. This is the perfect length. I've included a bonus day at the end during which you may want to go online and purchase an extended diary. Or start your own.

The sections are set up so you can balance the input of food against the output of what you burn.

Stuff in vs stuff out.

The '*stuff in*' box has breakfast, lunch, snacks and supper. Plus an area to note your drinks. Don't forget to not add cream or sugar, then step away from fruit juices and fizzy stuff.

Try to keep the snacks box empty. Avoid eating to fill emotional holes and avoid nibbly procrastination. Beware of 50/50 poisons.

Note how many hours you spend sat each day. Get this number down as the days pass.

The '*stuff out*' box has two columns. One for cardiovascular workouts. One for strength and core. Include housework, gardening, shopping, sex and anything that burns calories. Do more and more as the days pass.

I've included a section for '**sneaky extra activities**'. Fill this up for extra smug points.

For your daily total balance the cals in and the cals out. Fill your balance box. Most of us have a 2000 calorie daily allowance as our baseline. Down to 1500 if you are small woman, though 2500 if you are a big bloke.

Are you in positive balance for the day (an **oink** day) or negative (a **yay** day to make you go hooray)?

* * *

Your brain will work better if you complete the three daily psychological prompts.

- *This got in my way* …a note on your obstacles and stepping stones you face.

- *I'm pleased with this* …anything you did well, or if fortune smiled on you today.

- *One happy thought* …this can be anything. Something you are grateful for. Perhaps someone you love or who loves you.

Skinny Genes

Progress Diary

Monday

Day 1

today's goals: ....

stuff in

breakfast:	lunch:	snacks:	supper:

drinks:

hours sat not moving (tv, car, sofa) =

cals in =

vs

stuff out

cardio	strength and core
(walk / bike / run / swim)	(gym / yoga / sit-ups / planks)

sneaky extra activities:

cals out =

This got in my way today:

I'm pleased with this:

One happy thought:

balance (in -out) =

oink or yay?

Tuesday
Day 2

today's goals: ....

stuff in

breakfast:	lunch:	snacks:	supper:

drinks:

hours sat not moving (tv, car, sofa) =

cals in =

vs

stuff out

cardio

(walk / bike / run / swim)

strength and core

(gym / yoga / sit-ups / planks)

sneaky extra activities:

cals out =

This got in my way today:

I'm pleased with this:

One happy thought:

balance (in -out) =

oink or yay?

Wednesday

Day 3

today's goals: ....

stuff in

breakfast:	lunch:	snacks:	supper:

drinks:

hours sat not moving (tv, car, sofa) =

cals in =

vs

stuff out

cardio	strength and core
(walk / bike / run / swim)	(gym / yoga / sit-ups / planks)

sneaky extra activities:

cals out =

This got in my way today:

I'm pleased with this:

One happy thought:

balance (in -out) =

oink or yay?

Thursday
Day 4

today's goals: ....

stuff in

breakfast:	lunch:	snacks:	supper:

drinks:

hours sat not moving (tv, car, sofa) =

cals in =

vs

stuff out

cardio	strength and core
(walk / bike / run / swim)	(gym / yoga / sit-ups / planks)

sneaky extra activities:

cals out =

This got in my way today:

I'm pleased with this:

One happy thought:

balance (in -out) =

oink or yay?

Friday
Day 5

today's goals: ....

---

stuff in

breakfast:	lunch:	snacks:	supper:

drinks:

hours sat not moving (tv, car, sofa) =

cals in =

---

vs

---

stuff out

cardio
(walk / bike / run / swim)

strength and core
(gym / yoga / sit-ups / planks)

_____   _____
_____   _____
_____   _____
_____   _____
_____   _____

sneaky extra activities:

cals out =

This got in my way today:
I'm pleased with this:
One happy thought:

balance (in -out) =

oink or yay?

Saturday
Day 6

today's goals: ....

stuff in

breakfast:	lunch:	snacks:	supper:

drinks:

hours sat not moving (tv, car, sofa) =

cals in =

vs

stuff out

cardio	strength and core
(walk / bike / run / swim)	(gym / yoga / sit-ups / planks)

sneaky extra activities:

cals out =

This got in my way today:

I'm pleased with this:

One happy thought:

balance (in -out) =

oink or yay?

Sunday
Day 7

today's goals: ....

stuff in

breakfast:	lunch:	snacks:	supper:

drinks:

hours sat not moving (tv, car, sofa) =

cals in =

vs

stuff out

cardio	strength and core
(walk / bike / run / swim)	(gym / yoga / sit-ups / planks)

sneaky extra activities:

cals out =

This got in my way today:

I'm pleased with this:

One happy thought:

balance (in -out) =

oink or yay?

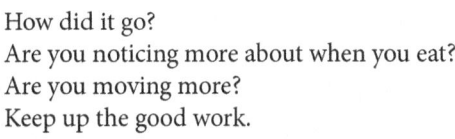

End of week one ...

How did it go?
Are you noticing more about when you eat?
Are you moving more?
Keep up the good work.

"We are what we repeatedly do. Excellence, there-fore, is not an act but a habit."

Aristotle (384 BC - 322 BC). Greek philosopher and scientist.

Monday
Day 8

today's goals: ....

stuff in

breakfast:	lunch:	snacks:	supper:

drinks:

hours sat not moving (tv, car, sofa) =

cals in =

vs

stuff out

cardio	strength and core
(walk / bike / run / swim)	(gym / yoga / sit-ups / planks)

sneaky extra activities:

cals out =

This got in my way today:

I'm pleased with this:

One happy thought:

balance (in -out) =

oink or yay?

Tuesday

Day 9

today's goals: ....

stuff in

breakfast:	lunch:	snacks:	supper:

drinks:

hours sat not moving (tv, car, sofa) =

cals in =

vs

stuff out

cardio	strength and core
(walk / bike / run / swim)	(gym / yoga / sit-ups / planks)

sneaky extra activities:

cals out =

This got in my way today:

I'm pleased with this:

One happy thought:

balance (in -out) =

oink or yay?

Wednesday
Day 10

today's goals: ....

stuff in

breakfast:	lunch:	snacks:	supper:

drinks:

hours sat not moving (tv, car, sofa) =

cals in =

vs

stuff out

cardio	strength and core
(walk / bike / run / swim)	(gym / yoga / sit-ups / planks)

sneaky extra activities:

cals out =

This got in my way today:

I'm pleased with this:

One happy thought:

balance (in -out) =

oink or yay?

Thursday

Day 11

today's goals: ....

stuff in

breakfast:	lunch:	snacks:	supper:

drinks:

hours sat not moving (tv, car, sofa) =

cals in =

vs

stuff out

cardio	strength and core
(walk / bike / run / swim)	(gym / yoga / sit-ups / planks)

sneaky extra activities:

cals out =

This got in my way today:

I'm pleased with this:

One happy thought:

balance (in -out) =

oink or yay?

Friday

Day 12

today's goals: ....

stuff in

breakfast:	lunch:	snacks:	supper:

drinks:

hours sat not moving (tv, car, sofa) =

cals in =

vs

stuff out

cardio

(walk / bike / run / swim)

strength and core

(gym / yoga / sit-ups / planks)

———————————
———————————
———————————
———————————
———————————

———————————
———————————
———————————
———————————
———————————

sneaky extra activities:

cals out =

This got in my way today:

I'm pleased with this:

One happy thought:

balance (in -out) =

oink or yay?

Saturday
Day 13

today's goals: ....

---

stuff in

breakfast:	lunch:	snacks:	supper:

drinks:

hours sat not moving (tv, car, sofa) =

cals in =

---

vs

---

stuff out

cardio	strength and core
(walk / bike / run / swim)	(gym / yoga / sit-ups / planks)

cardio
_____
_____
_____
_____
_____

strength and core
_____
_____
_____
_____

sneaky extra activities:

cals out =

This got in my way today:

I'm pleased with this:

One happy thought:

balance (in -out) =

oink or yay?

Sunday

Day 14

today's goals: ....

stuff in

breakfast:	lunch:	snacks:	supper:

drinks:

hours sat not moving (tv, car, sofa) =

cals in =

vs

stuff out

cardio

(walk / bike / run / swim)

strength and core

(gym / yoga / sit-ups / planks)

_____

_____

_____

_____

_____

_____

_____

_____

sneaky extra activities:

cals out =

This got in my way today:

I'm pleased with this:

One happy thought:

balance (in -out) =

oink or yay?

End of week two ...

How is it going so far?
Are some days easier than others?
That's ok. Roll with the punches.
Keep going.

"I've missed over 9,000 shots in my career.
I've lost almost 300 games.
26 times I've been trusted to take the game-win-
ning shot and missed.
I've failed over and over and over again in my life.
And that is why I succeed."

Michael Jordan (born February 17, 1963). Widely considered the greatest basketball player of all time.

Monday

Day 15

today's goals: ....

stuff in

breakfast:	lunch:	snacks:	supper:

drinks:

hours sat not moving (tv, car, sofa) =

cals in =

vs

stuff out

cardio

(walk / bike / run / swim)

strength and core

(gym / yoga / sit-ups / planks)

_____ _____

_____ _____

_____ _____

_____ _____

_____

sneaky extra activities:

cals out =

This got in my way today:

I'm pleased with this:

One happy thought:

balance (in -out) =

oink or yay?

Tuesday

Day 16

today's goals: ....

stuff in

breakfast:	lunch:	snacks:	supper:

drinks:

hours sat not moving (tv, car, sofa) =

cals in =

vs

stuff out

cardio

(walk / bike / run / swim)

strength and core

(gym / yoga / sit-ups / planks)

sneaky extra activities:

cals out =

This got in my way today:

I'm pleased with this:

One happy thought:

balance (in -out) =

oink or yay?

Wednesday
Day 17

today's goals: ....

stuff in

breakfast:	lunch:	snacks:	supper:

drinks:

hours sat not moving (tv, car, sofa) =

cals in =

vs

stuff out

cardio	strength and core
(walk / bike / run / swim)	(gym / yoga / sit-ups / planks)

sneaky extra activities:

cals out =

This got in my way today:

I'm pleased with this:

One happy thought:

balance (in -out) =

oink or yay?

Thursday

Day 18

today's goals: ....

stuff in

breakfast:	lunch:	snacks:	supper:

drinks:

hours sat not moving (tv, car, sofa) =

cals in =

vs

stuff out

cardio	strength and core
(walk / bike / run / swim)	(gym / yoga / sit-ups / planks)

sneaky extra activities:

cals out =

This got in my way today:

I'm pleased with this:

One happy thought:

balance (in -out) =

oink or yay?

Friday

Day 19

today's goals: ....

stuff in

breakfast:	lunch:	snacks:	supper:

drinks:

hours sat not moving (tv, car, sofa) =

cals in =

vs

stuff out

cardio

(walk / bike / run / swim)

strength and core

(gym / yoga / sit-ups / planks)

_____   _____
_____   _____
_____   _____
_____   _____

sneaky extra activities:

cals out =

This got in my way today:

I'm pleased with this:

One happy thought:

balance (in -out) =

oink or yay?

Saturday

Day 20

today's goals: ....

stuff in

breakfast:	lunch:	snacks:	supper:

drinks:

hours sat not moving (tv, car, sofa) =

cals in =

vs

stuff out

cardio	strength and core
(walk / bike / run / swim)	(gym / yoga / sit-ups / planks)

sneaky extra activities:

cals out =

This got in my way today:

I'm pleased with this:

One happy thought:

balance (in -out) =

oink or yay?

Sunday
Day 21

today's goals: ....

stuff in

breakfast:	lunch:	snacks:	supper:

drinks:

hours sat not moving (tv, car, sofa) =

cals in =

vs

stuff out

cardio
(walk / bike / run / swim)

_____
_____
_____
_____
_____

strength and core
(gym / yoga / sit-ups / planks)

_____
_____
_____
_____

sneaky extra activities:

cals out =

This got in my way today:
I'm pleased with this:
One happy thought:

balance (in -out) =

oink or yay?

End of week three ...

Good tenacity.
Making better choices will shape your future.
Steer clear of temptations when you are tired.
Never go shopping when you are hungry.

"We can do anything we want to do if we stick to it long enough."

Helen Keller (1880 - 1968). American writer. Deaf and blind from 19 months.

Monday

Day 22

today's goals: ....

stuff in

breakfast:	lunch:	snacks:	supper:

drinks:

hours sat not moving (tv, car, sofa) =

cals in =

vs

stuff out

cardio	strength and core
(walk / bike / run / swim)	(gym / yoga / sit-ups / planks)

sneaky extra activities:

cals out =

This got in my way today:

I'm pleased with this:

One happy thought:

balance (in -out) =

oink or yay?

Tuesday
Day 23

today's goals: ....

stuff in

breakfast:	lunch:	snacks:	supper:

drinks:

hours sat not moving (tv, car, sofa) =

cals in =

vs

stuff out

cardio

(walk / bike / run / swim)

strength and core

(gym / yoga / sit-ups / planks)

sneaky extra activities:

cals out =

This got in my way today:

I'm pleased with this:

One happy thought:

balance (in -out) =

oink or yay?

Wednesday
Day 24

today's goals: ....

stuff in

breakfast:	lunch:	snacks:	supper:

drinks:

hours sat not moving (tv, car, sofa) =

cals in =

vs

stuff out

cardio

(walk / bike / run / swim)

strength and core

(gym / yoga / sit-ups / planks)

_____

_____

_____

_____

_____

_____

_____

_____

sneaky extra activities:

cals out =

This got in my way today:

I'm pleased with this:

One happy thought:

balance (in -out) =

oink or yay?

Thursday

Day 25

today's goals: ....

stuff in

breakfast:	lunch:	snacks:	supper:

drinks:

hours sat not moving (tv, car, sofa) =

cals in =

vs

stuff out

cardio	strength and core
(walk / bike / run / swim)	(gym / yoga / sit-ups / planks)

sneaky extra activities:

cals out =

This got in my way today:

I'm pleased with this:

One happy thought:

balance (in -out) =

oink or yay?

Friday
Day 26

today's goals: ....

stuff in

breakfast:	lunch:	snacks:	supper:

drinks:

hours sat not moving (tv, car, sofa) =

cals in =

vs

stuff out

cardio	strength and core
(walk / bike / run / swim)	(gym / yoga / sit-ups / planks)

sneaky extra activities:

cals out =

This got in my way today:

I'm pleased with this:

One happy thought:

balance (in -out) =

oink or yay?

Saturday

Day 27

today's goals: ....

stuff in

breakfast:	lunch:	snacks:	supper:

drinks:

hours sat not moving (tv, car, sofa) =

cals in =

vs

stuff out

cardio

(walk / bike / run / swim)

strength and core

(gym / yoga / sit-ups / planks)

_____

_____

_____

_____

_____

_____

_____

_____

sneaky extra activities:

cals out =

This got in my way today:

I'm pleased with this:

One happy thought:

balance (in -out) =

oink or yay?

Sunday

Day 28

today's goals: ....

stuff in

breakfast:	lunch:	snacks:	supper:

drinks:

hours sat not moving (tv, car, sofa) =

cals in =

vs

stuff out

cardio

(walk / bike / run / swim)

strength and core

(gym / yoga / sit-ups / planks)

_____

_____

_____

_____

_____

_____

_____

_____

sneaky extra activities:

cals out =

This got in my way today:

I'm pleased with this:

One happy thought:

balance (in -out) =

oink or yay?

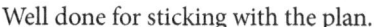

End of week four ...

Well done for sticking with the plan.
You are halfway through the days it takes to ingrain a habit.
Every day builds on the last.
Don't forget sneaky exercise moves.

"If you're going through hell, keep going."

By unknown (often misattributed to Winston Churchill).

Monday

Day 29

today's goals: ....

---

stuff in

breakfast:	lunch:	snacks:	supper:

drinks:

hours sat not moving (tv, car, sofa) =

cals in =

vs

stuff out

cardio	strength and core
(walk / bike / run / swim)	(gym / yoga / sit-ups / planks)

sneaky extra activities:

cals out =

This got in my way today:

I'm pleased with this:

One happy thought:

balance (in -out) =

oink or yay?

Tuesday

Day 30

today's goals: ....

stuff in

breakfast:	lunch:	snacks:	supper:

drinks:

hours sat not moving (tv, car, sofa) =

cals in =

vs

stuff out

cardio	strength and core
(walk / bike / run / swim)	(gym / yoga / sit-ups / planks)

sneaky extra activities:

cals out =

This got in my way today:

I'm pleased with this:

One happy thought:

balance (in -out) =

oink or yay?

Wednesday
Day 31

today's goals: ....

stuff in

breakfast:	lunch:	snacks:	supper:

drinks:

hours sat not moving (tv, car, sofa) =

cals in =

vs

stuff out

cardio

(walk / bike / run / swim)

strength and core

(gym / yoga / sit-ups / planks)

sneaky extra activities:

cals out =

This got in my way today:

I'm pleased with this:

One happy thought:

balance (in -out) =

oink or yay?

Thursday

Day 32

today's goals: ....

---

stuff in

breakfast:	lunch:	snacks:	supper:

drinks:

hours sat not moving (tv, car, sofa) =

cals in =

vs

stuff out

cardio	strength and core
(walk / bike / run / swim)	(gym / yoga / sit-ups / planks)

sneaky extra activities:

cals out =

This got in my way today:

I'm pleased with this:

One happy thought:

balance (in -out) =

oink or yay?

Friday

Day 33

today's goals: ....

stuff in

breakfast: | lunch: | snacks: | supper:

drinks:

hours sat not moving (tv, car, sofa) =

cals in =

vs

stuff out

cardio

(walk / bike / run / swim)

strength and core

(gym / yoga / sit-ups / planks)

_____

_____

_____

_____

_____

_____

_____

_____

sneaky extra activities:

cals out =

This got in my way today:

I'm pleased with this:

One happy thought:

balance (in -out) =

oink or yay?

Saturday

Day 34

today's goals: ....

stuff in

breakfast:	lunch:	snacks:	supper:

drinks:

hours sat not moving (tv, car, sofa) =

cals in =

vs

stuff out

cardio

(walk / bike / run / swim)

strength and core

(gym / yoga / sit-ups / planks)

sneaky extra activities:

cals out =

This got in my way today:

I'm pleased with this:

One happy thought:

balance (in -out) =

oink or yay?

Sunday
Day 35

today's goals: ....

stuff in

breakfast:	lunch:	snacks:	supper:

drinks:

hours sat not moving (tv, car, sofa) =

cals in =

vs

stuff out

cardio	strength and core
(walk / bike / run / swim)	(gym / yoga / sit-ups / planks)

sneaky extra activities:

cals out =

This got in my way today:

I'm pleased with this:

One happy thought:

balance (in -out) =

oink or yay?

End of week five ...

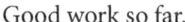

Good work so far.
I hope you are seeing the results of your efforts.
Stick at it.
Have you tried to see how long you can last without food
yet? The hungry days.

"Was mich nicht umbringt, macht mich stärker."
What does not kill me, makes me stronger.

Friedrich Wilhelm Nietzsche (1844 - 1900). German philosopher.

Monday
Day 36

today's goals: ....

stuff in

breakfast:	lunch:	snacks:	supper:

drinks:

hours sat not moving (tv, car, sofa) =

cals in =

vs

stuff out

cardio

(walk / bike / run / swim)

strength and core

(gym / yoga / sit-ups / planks)

———————————
———————————
———————————
———————————
———————————

———————————
———————————
———————————
———————————
———————————

sneaky extra activities:

cals out =

This got in my way today:

I'm pleased with this:

One happy thought:

balance (in -out) =

oink or yay?

Tuesday

Day 37

today's goals: ....

stuff in

| breakfast: | lunch: | snacks: | supper: |

drinks:

hours sat not moving (tv, car, sofa) =

| cals in = |

vs

stuff out

| cardio | strength and core |
| (walk / bike / run / swim) | (gym / yoga / sit-ups / planks) |

sneaky extra activities:

| cals out = |

This got in my way today:

I'm pleased with this:

One happy thought:

| balance (in -out) = |

oink or yay?

Wednesday

Day 38

today's goals: ....

stuff in

breakfast:	lunch:	snacks:	supper:

drinks:

hours sat not moving (tv, car, sofa) =

cals in =

vs

stuff out

cardio	strength and core
(walk / bike / run / swim)	(gym / yoga / sit-ups / planks)

sneaky extra activities:

cals out =

This got in my way today:

I'm pleased with this:

One happy thought:

balance (in -out) =

oink or yay?

Thursday

Day 39

today's goals: ....

---

stuff in

breakfast:	lunch:	snacks:	supper:

drinks:

hours sat not moving (tv, car, sofa) =

cals in =

vs

stuff out

cardio	strength and core
(walk / bike / run / swim)	(gym / yoga / sit-ups / planks)

sneaky extra activities:

cals out =

This got in my way today:

I'm pleased with this:

One happy thought:

balance (in -out) =

oink or yay?

Friday

Day 40

today's goals: ....

stuff in

breakfast:	lunch:	snacks:	supper:

drinks:

hours sat not moving (tv, car, sofa) =

cals in =

vs

stuff out

cardio

(walk / bike / run / swim)

strength and core

(gym / yoga / sit-ups / planks)

sneaky extra activities:

cals out =

This got in my way today:

I'm pleased with this:

One happy thought:

balance (in -out) =

oink or yay?

Saturday

Day 41

today's goals: ....

stuff in

breakfast:	lunch:	snacks:	supper:

drinks:

hours sat not moving (tv, car, sofa) =

cals in =

vs

stuff out

cardio	strength and core
(walk / bike / run / swim)	(gym / yoga / sit-ups / planks)

sneaky extra activities:

cals out =

This got in my way today:

I'm pleased with this:

One happy thought:

balance (in -out) =

oink or yay?

Sunday
Day 42

today's goals: ....

stuff in

breakfast:	lunch:	snacks:	supper:

drinks:

hours sat not moving (tv, car, sofa) =

cals in =

vs

stuff out

cardio	strength and core
(walk / bike / run / swim)	(gym / yoga / sit-ups / planks)

sneaky extra activities:

cals out =

This got in my way today:

I'm pleased with this:

One happy thought:

balance (in -out) =

oink or yay?

End of week six ...

I'm pleased that you are still filling your journal.
Tinkering with what we do brings great results.
Have you made an effort with your strength and muscles?
This is often overlooked.
I hope you are getting enough good quality sleep.

"To improve is to change, so to be perfect is to have changed often."

Sir Winston Churchill (1874 - 1965). British statesman.

Monday

Day 43

today's goals: ....

stuff in

breakfast:	lunch:	snacks:	supper:

drinks:

hours sat not moving (tv, car, sofa) =

cals in =

vs

stuff out

cardio

(walk / bike / run / swim)

strength and core

(gym / yoga / sit-ups / planks)

sneaky extra activities:

cals out =

This got in my way today:

I'm pleased with this:

One happy thought:

balance (in -out) =

oink or yay?

Tuesday
Day 44

today's goals: ....

stuff in

breakfast: | lunch: | snacks: | supper:

drinks:

hours sat not moving (tv, car, sofa) =

cals in =

vs

stuff out

cardio

(walk / bike / run / swim)

strength and core

(gym / yoga / sit-ups / planks)

_____

_____

_____

_____

_____

sneaky extra activities:

cals out =

This got in my way today:

I'm pleased with this:

One happy thought:

balance (in -out) =

oink or yay?

Wednesday
Day 45

today's goals: ....

---

stuff in

breakfast:	lunch:	snacks:	supper:

drinks:

hours sat not moving (tv, car, sofa) =

cals in =

vs

stuff out

cardio	strength and core
(walk / bike / run / swim)	(gym / yoga / sit-ups / planks)

sneaky extra activities:

cals out =

This got in my way today:

I'm pleased with this:

One happy thought:

balance (in -out) =

oink or yay?

Thursday

Day 46

today's goals: ....

stuff in

breakfast:	lunch:	snacks:	supper:

drinks:

hours sat not moving (tv, car, sofa) =

cals in =

vs

stuff out

cardio	strength and core
(walk / bike / run / swim)	(gym / yoga / sit-ups / planks)

sneaky extra activities:

cals out =

This got in my way today:

I'm pleased with this:

One happy thought:

balance (in -out) =

oink or yay?

Friday
Day 47

today's goals: ....

stuff in

breakfast:	lunch:	snacks:	supper:

drinks:

hours sat not moving (tv, car, sofa) =

cals in =

vs

stuff out

cardio

(walk / bike / run / swim)

strength and core

(gym / yoga / sit-ups / planks)

sneaky extra activities:

cals out =

This got in my way today:

I'm pleased with this:

One happy thought:

balance (in -out) =

oink or yay?

Saturday

Day 48

today's goals: ....

stuff in

breakfast:	lunch:	snacks:	supper:

drinks:

hours sat not moving (tv, car, sofa) =

cals in =

vs

stuff out

cardio

(walk / bike / run / swim)

strength and core

(gym / yoga / sit-ups / planks)

sneaky extra activities:

cals out =

This got in my way today:

I'm pleased with this:

One happy thought:

balance (in -out) =

oink or yay?

Sunday

Day 49

today's goals: ....

stuff in

| breakfast: | lunch: | snacks: | supper: |

drinks:

hours sat not moving (tv, car, sofa) =

cals in =

vs

stuff out

| cardio | strength and core |
| (walk / bike / run / swim) | (gym / yoga / sit-ups / planks) |

sneaky extra activities:

cals out =

This got in my way today:

I'm pleased with this:

One happy thought:

balance (in -out) =

oink or yay?

End of week seven ...

Great work to still be here.
I hope you are pleased with yourself.
Are you on you behind for too many hours in a day?
Get out of the front door more often. Even in awful weather.

"I have insecurities of course, but I don't hang out with anyone who points them out to me."

Adele (born 5 May 1988). English singer-songwriter.

Monday

Day 50

today's goals: ....

stuff in

breakfast:	lunch:	snacks:	supper:

drinks:

hours sat not moving (tv, car, sofa) =

cals in =

vs

stuff out

cardio	strength and core
(walk / bike / run / swim)	(gym / yoga / sit-ups / planks)

sneaky extra activities:

cals out =

This got in my way today:

I'm pleased with this:

One happy thought:

balance (in -out) =

oink or yay?

Tuesday
Day 51

today's goals: ....

stuff in

breakfast:	lunch:	snacks:	supper:

drinks:

hours sat not moving (tv, car, sofa) =

cals in =

vs

stuff out

cardio	strength and core
(walk / bike / run / swim)	(gym / yoga / sit-ups / planks)

sneaky extra activities:

cals out =

This got in my way today:

I'm pleased with this:

One happy thought:

balance (in -out) =

oink or yay?

Wednesday

Day 52

today's goals: ....

stuff in

breakfast:	lunch:	snacks:	supper:

drinks:

hours sat not moving (tv, car, sofa) =

cals in =

vs

stuff out

cardio	strength and core
(walk / bike / run / swim)	(gym / yoga / sit-ups / planks)

sneaky extra activities:

cals out =

This got in my way today:

I'm pleased with this:

One happy thought:

balance (in -out) =

oink or yay?

Thursday
Day 53

today's goals: ....

stuff in

breakfast:	lunch:	snacks:	supper:

drinks:

hours sat not moving (tv, car, sofa) =

cals in =

vs

stuff out

cardio

(walk / bike / run / swim)

strength and core

(gym / yoga / sit-ups / planks)

_____

_____

_____

_____

_____

_____

_____

_____

sneaky extra activities:

cals out =

This got in my way today:

I'm pleased with this:

One happy thought:

balance (in -out) =

oink or yay?

Friday

Day 54

today's goals: ....

stuff in

breakfast:	lunch:	snacks:	supper:

drinks:

hours sat not moving (tv, car, sofa) =

cals in =

vs

stuff out

cardio	strength and core
(walk / bike / run / swim)	(gym / yoga / sit-ups / planks)

sneaky extra activities:

cals out =

This got in my way today:

I'm pleased with this:

One happy thought:

balance (in -out) =

oink or yay?

Saturday

Day 55

today's goals: ....

stuff in

| breakfast: | lunch: | snacks: | supper: |

drinks:

hours sat not moving (tv, car, sofa) =

cals in =

vs

stuff out

cardio

(walk / bike / run / swim)

strength and core

(gym / yoga / sit-ups / planks)

_____

_____

_____

_____

_____

_____

_____

_____

_____

_____

sneaky extra activities:

cals out =

This got in my way today:

I'm pleased with this:

One happy thought:

balance (in -out) =

oink or yay?

Sunday

Day 56

today's goals: ....

stuff in

breakfast:	lunch:	snacks:	supper:

drinks:

hours sat not moving (tv, car, sofa) =

cals in =

vs

stuff out

cardio

(walk / bike / run / swim)

strength and core

(gym / yoga / sit-ups / planks)

sneaky extra activities:

cals out =

This got in my way today:

I'm pleased with this:

One happy thought:

balance (in -out) =

oink or yay?

End of week eight ...

How is the naked mirror check? Improving?
It takes just over sixty days to get your new success habits.
Well done on being nearly there.
If you've found this helpful - a longer version is for sale
...(shameless plug).

"The best time to plant a tree was 20 years ago. The second best time is now."

Chinese Proverb

Monday

Day 57

today's goals: ....

stuff in

| breakfast: | lunch: | snacks: | supper: |

drinks:

hours sat not moving (tv, car, sofa) =

cals in =

vs

stuff out

| cardio | strength and core |
| (walk / bike / run / swim) | (gym / yoga / sit-ups / planks) |

sneaky extra activities:

cals out =

This got in my way today:

I'm pleased with this:

One happy thought:

balance (in -out) =

oink or yay?

Tuesday

Day 58

today's goals: ....

stuff in

breakfast:	lunch:	snacks:	supper:

drinks:

hours sat not moving (tv, car, sofa) =

cals in =

vs

stuff out

cardio	strength and core
(walk / bike / run / swim)	(gym / yoga / sit-ups / planks)

sneaky extra activities:

cals out =

This got in my way today:

I'm pleased with this:

One happy thought:

balance (in -out) =

oink or yay?

Wednesday

Day 59

today's goals: ....

stuff in

breakfast:	lunch:	snacks:	supper:

drinks:

hours sat not moving (tv, car, sofa) =

cals in =

vs

stuff out

cardio	strength and core
(walk / bike / run / swim)	(gym / yoga / sit-ups / planks)

sneaky extra activities:

cals out =

This got in my way today:

I'm pleased with this:

One happy thought:

balance (in -out) =

oink or yay?

Thursday

Day 60

today's goals: ....

stuff in

breakfast:	lunch:	snacks:	supper:

drinks:

hours sat not moving (tv, car, sofa) =

cals in =

vs

stuff out

cardio	strength and core
(walk / bike / run / swim)	(gym / yoga / sit-ups / planks)

sneaky extra activities:

cals out =

This got in my way today:

I'm pleased with this:

One happy thought:

balance (in -out) =

oink or yay?

Friday

Day 61

today's goals: ....

stuff in

breakfast:	lunch:	snacks:	supper:

drinks:

hours sat not moving (tv, car, sofa) =

cals in =

vs

stuff out

cardio

(walk / bike / run / swim)

strength and core

(gym / yoga / sit-ups / planks)

sneaky extra activities:

cals out =

This got in my way today:

I'm pleased with this:

One happy thought:

balance (in -out) =

oink or yay?

Well done for finishing the diary. I hope that your new habits will prove really helpful in your beach-ready body quest.

If you would find it useful, there are follow-on diaries available for sale at:
Amazon.com
brainsolutions.co.uk

Check out brainsolutions.co.uk for more titles by Dr Phil Harley
coming soon ...

BetterDay - stress management for busy people

Do it, *do it,* **DO IT!** - a Procastinator's Guide to World Domination

Beginners guide to running

If you enjoyed this, I would very much appreciate you leaving feedback on Amazon.

Sign up today at **brainsolutions.co.uk** for:

20 daily tips - FREE daily emails to give you a boost in your Waist Management

About the author

Dr Harley lives and works in the South of the UK with his family.

In his spare time he reads more about running than is probably good for him.

He's told he should get out more (though he obviously thinks that means on the trails).

A family doctor with twenty years experience and a specialist in weight management.

Sign up for his free 20 daily tips email if you'd like to more tips on how to manage your waist.

If you have feedback, comments, questions or suggestions, please email drphil@brainsolutions.co.uk

www.ingramcontent.com/pod-product-compliance
Lightning Source LLC
Chambersburg PA
CBHW070851180526
45168CB00005B/1767